GOOD NEWS FOR THE ALPHABET KIDS

Other books by Michael Sichel

Bitter-Sweet Profits
The truth behind the diabetic drug industry
and the success of a non-drug method that reverses Diabetes II

Mercury, Man and Medicine
The history, the results and the answers
with Alan E. Moses

Janelle,

Having met you in College, your warmth and kindness were never an effort - they were simply who you are and always will be. May this book's knowledge be shared with others as you continue your life of gratitude and giving. You were always in my thoughts and never forgotten. Blessings of Health, Happiness and Harmony on this journey called life!

Sending Love & Positive Vibes!!!

GOOD NEWS FOR THE ALPHABET KIDS

How to reverse learning & behavioural disorders without drugs

Michael Sichel DO ND PhD
author of
How to beat hyperactivity without drugs

NUTRITIONAL SECTION by Greta Sichel DO ND

Good news for the alphabet kids!

How to reverse learning & behavioural disorders without drugs

First published March 2004
Revised and updated edition February 2005

ISBN 1 74011 031 5

Published by Bookbound Publishing
PO Box 309, Ourimbah, NSW 2258, Australia
FreeCall 1800 628 058 (Australia only)
Int'l phone +612 4362 8058
info@bookbound.com.au

Michael Sichel is available in Australia for presentations on children's health, hyperactive behaviour and learning problems related to ADD/ADHD or ASD.

Fountaindale Clinic, Box 5054, Chittaway Bay, NSW 2261

Telephone (02) 4362 2458, Facsimile (02) 4362 8112

Email sichel@hotkey.net.au

"The Curse does not come without a Cause ..."

Proverbs 26:2

The 'why' behind our children's woes

Be prepared to be shocked and angered by the recent exposures

Functional Medicine Doctors and Naturopaths share a passion to find the reasons why a person with a problem has come to consult them. They have found that multiple factors are usually behind every hurting person. They do not believe that some magic pill will bring true healing. Nor do they blame what must be incredibly fast genetic factors or elusive 'Scarlet Pimpernel' viruses for *every* otherwise unidentified cause of a rapidly advancing pandemic.

They do know, however, that you must find the true cause or causes before you can reverse the results.

Some 40 pages of this book deal with the extremely controversial multiple reasons behind our modern epidemic of child problems. What you will read will shock and anger you. But below are brief statements taken directly from the current United States Congress investigation (now in its third year) into all the childhood learning and behaviour problems, from serious regressive autism to a mildly slow learner with attention difficulties.

Incredible as it may seem, the medically qualified Senators[1] on this Senate Committee have found the US health industry regulators, pharmaceutical companies and certain branches of modern medicine responsible. Not only responsible, but (in some cases) deliberately falsifying data to protect themselves, deliberately allowing highly dangerous substances to be given to our children, despite warnings from some of their own scientists!

Institutions like the Centres for Disease Control (CDC) and the Food and Drug Administration (FDA) have been found in serious neglect of their fiduciary duty to the people who trust them – in this case, the parents. Unfortunately, these American regulators heavily influence the Australian Therapeutics Goods Authority (TGA), who, it appears, open wide the doors on well-oiled hinges, to the same medical practices.[2]

Careful investigation has found these causes relate to as high as 80% of our children's learning and behaviour problems. One of the major problems is mercury preservative (thimerosal aka thiomersal[3,4,5]) in vaccines. CDC scientists wrote a falsified report that down-played this concern. A concern that applied to millions of American, Australian, British and many other nations' children. This was discovered through the use of the Freedom of Information Act. The Chief Writer then left the CDC to work for the drug company that produced mercury containing preservatives!

From a letter[6] written by Dr Dave Weldon, Member of Congress to the Director of the CDC, Dr Julie Gerberding, October 31, 2003: "I have reviewed the transcripts of a discussion at Simpsonwood, GA between the author (of a false study), various CDC employees and vaccine industry representatives."

This discussion was behind closed doors, but recorded. Here are just some of the dark secrets they discussed:

- We can push and pull this data anyway we want.
- There was really no need to do this study, we could have predicted the outcomes. **(*Editor*: the outcomes were these: a direct correlation was found between amount of exposure to mercury in vaccines and the risk and severity of the disorder.)**
- I will not give thimerosal (mercury containing vaccine preservative) to my grandson until I find out what is going on here.
- This information should be kept confidential and embargoed.
- The significant association with language delay is quite large (study Chief Writer).

1 D Sam Weldon, www.reform.house.gov/WHR

2 See Prevnar Investigations and www.909shot.com

3 Rashid Buttar DO FAAPM, American Board of Clinical Metal Toxicology (Chairman), testimony before Congress, May6, 2004

4 Eli Lilly, documented on their own letterhead as far back as July 1991, clearly states that thimerosal is a "product containing a chemical known to the State of California to cause birth defects or other reproductive harm". Yet, Eli Lily continues to use thimerosal in the manufacturing process for vaccines.

5 June11, 2004 – Thimerosal, the ethylmercury-based preservative found in childhood vaccines, can increase the risk of autism-like damage in mice, according to a report published online on June 8, 2004 in advance of publication in *Molecular Psychiatry*.

6 Copy held by author – see reference 82, page 271.

'I am now convinced that in ways we do not yet understand, the behaviour of both the allergic child and adult can be altered and modified as dramatically by foods as it can be altered by drugs.'

John W. Gerrard
Professor of Pediatrics, University of Saskatchewan, Canada

'The research has shown that diet definitely affects some children. Symptoms which may change include those seen in Attention Deficit Disorder (ADD) and Attention Deficit Hyperactive Disorder (ADHD), sleep problems, physical symptoms ... [and] particularly changes in mood.'

J.Breakey
Journal of Paediatric Child Health, June 1997

Dietery replacement in pre-school hyperactive boys

'More than half the subjects exhibited reliable improvement in behaviour and negligible placebo effects. In addition, several nonbehavioral variables tended to improve ... particularly halitosis, night awakenings and latency to sleep onset.'

B.Kaplan et al
Pediatrics, 1989 Vol 83

'150 of 200 children (75%) improved in an open trial of a diet free of synthetic food coloring.'

K.S. Rowe and K.J. Rowe
Double-blind, placebo controlled, repeated-measures study
Journal of Pediatrics, November 1994

The information in this book is based on the training, personal experiences and research of the author. It is intended for educational purposes and is not meant to diagnose, prescribe or replace medical care. Mention of any research organisation or individual researcher should in no way be construed as an endorsement of this book or any of the techniques herein.

Because each person and situation is unique, the author and the publisher urge the reader to check with a qualified health professional before using any procedure for which there is any question of appropriateness. It is a sign of wisdom, not cowardice, to seek a second or third opinion.

The publisher does not advocate the use of any particular health treatment, but believes the information presented in this book should be available to the public.

The author and the publisher cannot accept responsibility nor will be held responsible in any way or for any actions taken by the reader upon reading the material in this book. If the reader decides to take any action as a result of reading this book, he or she agrees to do so entirely at their own risk and responsibility and agrees to completely indemnify the author and publisher against any legal responsibility or compensation for harm or loss.

NOTE

A few specific brandname natural medicines and nutrients used by the author and mentioned in this book are only available in Australia. However, their equivalent can be found in most other countries.

Dedication

This book is dedicated to the tens of thousands of perplexed and suffering parents and their children who drifted, or stormed, into another world, the world of ADHD & all autism spectrum disorders – the Land of Question Marks. Many of you have tried all kinds of therapies. This book helps to identify and repair the *cause(s)* of your child's problems.

Sincere thanks to all who helped build this book

To my wife and helpmate Greta, whose love and patience always endured. To my daughter Monika, for her determination to 'read the MS', despite her very busy family life, a counselling course and her church work with husband Paul.

To editor Jane Derby, who unwittingly caused me to rewrite the whole book.

To my publisher Eric Hook, who sometimes wondered if I was either dead, lost or had migrated.

To Gairden Cooke and Steven Cooper, Disney animators/cartoonists, for arranging and drawing the happy little guy on the cover.

To Dr Archie Kalokerinos whose determination and courage in the face of medical and government persecution has been an inspiration. Surely, his work for innocent parent/carer victims of Shaken Baby Syndrome will one day make an epic book and movie.

And to the other fighters in that and other causes – Dr Mark Donohue, Dr Vera Scheibner, Dr Robyn Cosford, Dr Joachim Fluhrer and Meryl Dorey of AVN.

And to all who gave time to read the manuscript and improved it – Chris Porter PhD DO, Terry Hinton, Geoff Baker PhD and all others who gave advice.

But, above all, to the Great Physician who lived among us for a while. The Man who would lead us into all truth, brought us hope and showed us what love means. Rejected by some, welcomed by others. His was a life that has changed our world for the better.

Foreword

In this book, Michael Sichel provides an overview of the many issues surrounding attention deficit disorder (ADD), attention deficit hyperactivity disorder (ADHD) and all autistic spectrum disorders (ASDs). Michael has drawn on years of experience, knowledge and skill as a health professional, to reaffirm that the fundamental requirement for good health is good food.

This book encourages us to take a fresh look at the potential cumulative impact of diet, antibiotics and vaccination on the immune systems of our children, and ultimately on their behaviour. It reflects modern understandings of abnormal gastrointestinal bacteria and other organisms that now point to a revival of the old concept of *disease origins* and examines the chain of events that can lead to systemic candidiasis, chronic dysfunction of the digestive tract and, in turn, ASD and ADD/ADHD.

Overall, I find this book to be a balanced and educated consideration of issues that are vital to our children and to ourselves, and to the community in which we live.

Michael Sichel is to be congratulated, and thanked, for the effort involved and the skill so obviously displayed.

Dr Archie Kalokerinos MB BS AOM
Author of the best-selling book *Every Second Child*

Synopsis of Chapters

Appendices

Use of the term 'ASD'

Autism Spectrum Disorder (ASD) has now become the term for a wide range of childhood problems[1] associated with the current international childhood epidemic of behaviour, development and learning issues, such as ADHD (Attention Deficit Hyperactive Disorder). For purposes of brevity, ASD in this book includes most of the problems that affect the mind/mental health of a child. The reasons are explained in the Treatment Chapter.

In 1990 only one or two per 10,000 children suffered from an autistic disorder. Today, more than one in 150 children suffer from regressive (late-onset) autism[2], plus hundreds of thousands more with lesser but often similar symptoms. (Website 'hits' for ADHD advice are now more than 55,000 *monthly*.)

'The Alphabet Children'

Generally, I do not believe in precisely labelling a child publicly – that is, when both parents and child and their family and associates know that Johnny has ODD (Opposition Defiant), ADHD, PDD (Pervasive Development), ADD (Attention Deficit) or NOS (Not Otherwise Specified – how would you like to be labelled *not otherwise specified*?) and others.

It can be too complex and confrontational and unfairly mark the child for life, but it is helpful in the clinical situation and for interaction with other practitioners. Also, for medical claims. However, for everyday use I believe that ASD should be either of two embracing terms: "Johnny has ASD", or, "Johnny is an Alphabet child" – which most kids seem to prefer. This way, he is one of tens of thousands, and far less menacing than being a comparative minority.

I also believe the 'D' in ASD should stand for 'Disease' and not for 'Disorder'. There are any number of definitions dealing with autism and autism spectrum disorders … all share a common element. They all define ASDs as a disorder.

The accepted definition of autism as a disorder can be traced to its origins, now discredited, as a psychiatric condition … implicit in this is that ASDs are a life-long condition. **Explicit is the understanding that the child is the disorder and disorders are usually for life, ie not curable**.

This concept is reflected in the supermarkets daily, where hyperactive 'Alphabet' children plainly stand out. Parents of such children are often grimly stared at, and sometimes told, "He needs a good whack", or "He needs discipline".

Somehow, the child or the parent, or both, 'get the blame'. This suits the pharmaceutical and medical industry fine. The need for a quick-fix drug solution becomes imperative. But, as you will find in the Causes Chapter, if there is anyone to blame – and make no mistake about it, there is – it is not the parents, nor their genes, and certainly not the children.

Also, ASDs are not necessarily incurable. Therefore, they are a disease and not a 'disorder/condition'. Autism is curable.[3] That fact does not suit the pharmo-med duo.[4] For them the concept 'autism is incurable' equals a lifelong customer, whereas a recovery means a lost customer. And if the profound disease of autism is curable, then its near relatives – Aspergers, ADHD, ADD, ODD, PDD (the 'Alphabet Children') – should also be curable.

And they are!

NOTE: Throughout this book, the child, unless otherwise named, is usually described as a boy ('he' or 'him') – not just for ease of writing, but because eighty out of every one hundred ASD children are boys.

Author's Foreword

"A truth's initial commotion is directly proportional to how deeply the lie was believed ... When a well-packaged web of lies has been sold gradually to the masses over generations, the truth will seem utterly preposterous and its speaker, a raving lunatic."

Dresden James

At one weary point while writing this book a mother phoned me, crying. She said, "I don't know how to thank you enough, you have given us our son back." His kindergarten teacher had also cried, she said – with joy. One needs no greater spur than that.

That has been my chief motivation to keep going. Grateful parents and also grateful children, plus the vision of thousands 'out there' who still struggle.

In this book you will read the stories of Brock (3), Jordon (3), Richard (3), Emily (5), Joshua (5), Nicolle (7), Billy (8), Matthew (9), Luke (12) and others as old as 24 – who all came back from their own varied but pervasive 'black holes' of autism spectrum disorders and hyperactivity. And they came back without medical drugs, or no longer needed medical drugs.[5] They came back, paradoxically, not with brain drugs but by treating gastro-intestinal conditions, nutritional deficiencies and sometimes, toxic metal contamination, using the same methods later described by the Harvard University study of 400 ASD children in 2002.[6]

They are just a few of the many clients that have been treated successfully at our clinic, without drugs.

Not only did the shadows lift for these dear little children, but of course, for their parents.

I thought that the best way for you to understand the successful non-drug functional medicine approach to autism spectrum disease, is via detailed anecdotes from our clinic and other experts in the field. Therefore, some of these stories make up Chapter Six of this book and include the medical reasons for the results obtained.

Of course, this has to be supported by science. And it is now supported by large volumes of peer reviewed science, complete with the double-blind cross over studies considered so essential by orthodox medicine. You will find outstanding examples quoted in this book, plus a multitude of references from prestigious medical journals to substantiate our successes.

This large body of happy anecdotal evidence combined with standard science is compelling to those who will study with an open mind. (The unhappy part of this story is that, despite the anecdotal evidence and the references from recognised sources that non-drug functional medicine is successful in treating autism spectrum disorders, many authorities refuse to acknowledge this treatment exists or the benefits it provides. Reasons for this attitude will be explained in Part 1.)

Having said that, it is wise to remember that the pioneers of these treatments had NIL evidence of any kind that this treatment would prove successful. However, if they had stayed with the *status quo*, today there would be tens of thousands of children still 'lost' in the clouds and confusion of autism spectrum disorders. For the early researchers, multiple happy anecdotes were their only evidence to forge ahead.

So, in this book we present both the happy anecdotes and the compelling evidence from many famous institutions that include the Mayo Clinic, Utah University, Harvard, University of Sunderland (UK), and the Autism Research Institute. You will find the references as you go through the book, plus a Bibliography that includes reliable web-sites, as well as books and email addresses of ASD Groups parents can write to (which is often the most practical learning curve of all).

But best of all, as I have said, are the stories selected from the hundreds of children and their parents who have consulted with us over the years. Although every child reacts in an individual way, and every child has to be treated in a special way, there is a common thread that runs through 95% of ASD children. Because of that, you will surely recognise your own child in some of these stories.

Surveys indicate that 60% of Australians now use some form of alternative healthcare. Former Health Minister, Dr Michael Wooldridge, stated, "…we ignore other approaches and other models at our own risk and against community trends."

Three Universities now offer degree courses in naturopathy. In 2001, the La Trobe University in Victoria commenced Australia's first double degree course in Nursing and Naturopathy. A 1997 survey published in the Australian Medical Journal *revealed that 80% of the 488 doctors who responded had referred patients to alternative therapists; 20% of them had practiced or trained in one of these modalities.*

But you should question every practitioner you choose – whether he/she is a doctor, naturopath or specialises in some other modality. That practitioner may not be right for YOU. In our practice, we are disappointed if the client does not ask for evidence or questions treatment. ***Seek to become informed yourself.***

Introduction to this second book on ASD

This volume is about *all* the autism-connected 'Alphabet' diseases. The first book was named *How to beat hyperactivity without drugs*. Now I know, with absolute certainty, what I only suspected before. Most, if not all of the learning/behavioural problems are closely related.

The most researched ASD is autism. Autism has been the principle 'marker' or 'steady-line- on- the- graph', that has been used to track the severity of the current pandemic of 'mind' illness in our children. This is because autism numbers have been closely followed for some 40 years in several countries.

You will read more about this in the Causes Chapter. But autism used to be almost always a congenital event (the baby was born autistic). Today, the greatest number of autism is called 'regressive' (see panel graph). That is, the child is normal until typically nearly three years of age and then begins to lose previous skills and learning (speech, movement, affection etc). This sea-change began in the 1970's, but became a wave three years after the MMR vaccination began in USA (1978) and in the last decade became a tidal wave (see graph). The same occurred in the UK (1986) (exactly the number of years later when the mercury preserved MMR began in England). At the same time, all the many other ASD problems began to surge, and new ones appeared that had never been seen before. There is no total consensus, but altogether the 'Alphabet Diseases' usually include: ADHD, ODD, PDD, Retts Syndrome (RS), Aspergers (AS), Wilsons Disease, Smith-Magenis Syndrome (SMS), ADD and NOS (Not Specified Disorders).

Knowledge about the causes, treatment (and now – cures) of the current wide spread pandemic of childhood learning problems and illness is advancing in leaps and bounds. But the pandemic continues and increases, and new research from around the world still points to a combination of identifiable and *controllable* environmental factors as the major cause. Not primarily genetic[7,8] and not incurable – as the orthodox medical profession would have us believe.

Genetic causes could not suddenly become an epidemic

Autism and ASD rose exponentially in ten years (1991–2001). In Australia, there are now 17 new cases weekly – unheard of before 1996. In America, one in 140 children is now autistic, up from two or three in 10,000 twenty years ago.

Such 'sudden' changes can never be ascribed to normal mutational events. If genetics were the primary cause, every identical autistic twin would have an autistic sibling, only 60% have this occur. And even then the problem maybe traced to the same environmental cause to which they were both exposed.[9,10,11]

"There is increasing evidence that physical and chemical stresses to the cell, such as heat shock, chemical poisons and viral infections, tend to activate *Alu*[12] elements. The resultant gene reshuffling may be responsible for a variety of chronic diseases." (Dr Mae Wan Ho, Institute of Science in Society, UK 2003)

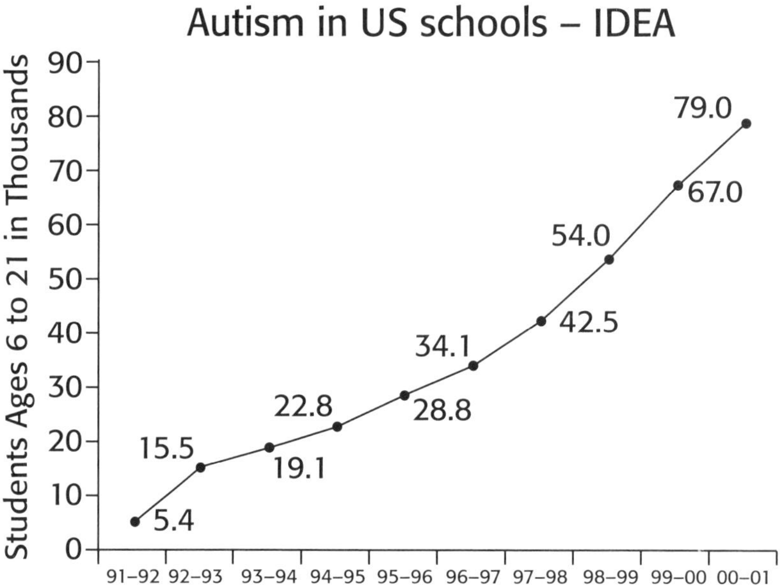

An Australian confirmation of this sharp upward curve was provided to me by a child care worker at one of my recent seminars. Anne told me that she had been in child care for 17 years and that she was amazed at the changes in that time, especially during the past six years. Her child groups have begun to hold more and more cases of allergy, asthma, autism and speech and hearing problems. Her organisation now employs a speech pathologist who is flat out trying to keep up with the demand. It's the same story at nine other centres in her region, she said.

To not stop the *causes* of this pandemic is equivalent to putting an ambulance down in the valley, instead of a fence at the top of the cliff!

The good news

Autism spectrum disorders (ASDs), the Alphabet Diseases – including a range of lesser behavioural and learning problems – are now being shown to be *functional* disorders (body functions affecting the brain's function) not brain damage and not primarily genetic, so much can be done to reverse and restore. That is what this book is about.

The body function problems mostly responsible for this affect centre on the immune system[13] and the gastro-intestinal tract. Several environmental factors plus individual inherited factors (all more or less reversible or controllable) are now known, but the major culprits have been identified as masked antibiotic and vaccine related damage – including the neurotoxin mercury used to preserve vaccines and also high lead and/or arsenic levels.

The types of ASD's, and numbers affected, have increased dramatically in the last 10 to 15 years (1:100 Australian children are now diagnosed with autism spectrum disorders). As we have mentioned, that period is the same time when so-called 'herd' immunisation began and includes the Hepatitis B decade when infants began to be 'shot' at birth or close thereafter, beginning the highest peak for autism ever seen. What is in these vaccines? How are they made? How efficient are they and what damage do they do? Are they all necessary? These vital questions are being asked today, and litigated with class-actions in the USA, Canada and United Kingdom. There is a great debate in the scientific community as to which vaccines cause damage and how much damage. The Appendix in this book covers these facts in depth.

Some of the causes

One child's reaction to environmental triggers varies from another's, depending on factors that often affect the efficiency of the child's immune system. These factors, in order of significance, include:

- Auto-immune reactions (often vaccine induced, usually masked but in my experience can be obvious in 26% of cases)[14];
- The burden of antibiotic treatments used for infections (themselves often triggered by immune weakening reactions to vaccination e.g. middle ear infections, now in 80% of children, represent 75% of 2nd visits to paediatricians,[15] yet were comparatively rare before 'herd' immunization began);
- Environmental chemical and heavy metal pollutants (e.g. mercury, in vaccines and maternal dental amalgams, lead and cadmium from industry, arsenic in the playground);
- Low levels of essential immune system nutrients;
- High levels of sugar in the diet – with subsequent disruption to immune and endocrine functions plus disruption of important mineral level ratios;

- Function of inherited immune defences, such as liver detoxification efficiency; and
- Birthing problems lie behind some autism and also ADD.

Antibiotics began to fail dramatically in the last 15 years, and children are the most susceptible, being 'the population segment with highest antibiotic resistance'.[16] Drug resistant bacteria and yeast forms are found in the gut of many of the children with ASDs, including ADHD. No wonder that children's immune systems have a fight on their hands!

Fortunately, as I have mentioned, most of the above problems are now repairable (and their causes discoverable through new pathology). Much of this therapy is nutritional plus special nutrient-enhanced remedies. "Children respond much faster and much more completely to nutritional therapy than do adults" to quote the famous paediatrician Leo Galland MD (*Superimmunity for Kids*, 1988). In my experience, the younger the child the faster the response.

It is necessary to point out that there are other very useful therapies for the learning, movement, interaction and speech problems of these children. They can be most helpful in a child who has already recovered significantly by treating the CAUSES. That child can be years behind in development, and now needs to 'catch-up'. Many of my clients had earlier used these adjunctive therapies for an answer, but were not satisfied. However, they went back to them after the basic problem had been 'fixed' by our functional medicine methods, to 'catch-up'.

For your own reading and research, please see the professional websites and organizations listed in the bibliography at end of this book. Meanwhile, you can now begin to reverse some or most of this damage.

The toxin-free nursery

Toxicologists have found that flame retardant chemicals (PBDEs), used in bedding, furniture and mattresses, can acculumulate in our bodies and cause mind altering problems like lowered intelligence, faulty memory, hyperactivity and other behavioural problems. The chemical build-up of PBDEs is as dangerous to our health and survival – or even more so – than the PCBs (polychlorinated biphenyls) and DDT that were found to accumulate in living cells and that were banned in the 1970s. Like the DDT by-products, if PBDEs were banned today, it would take many generations before the environment would be clear.

Both parents and their offspring are harmed by PBDEs which can invade the blood stream and cause chemical disruption. Wisely, the Europeans banned PBDE compounds when it was found that they accumulate in body cells and breast milk. The good news is that European women now have less fire retardant chemicals in their milk than before the ban. the bad news is that flame retardant chemicals are still not regulated in the United States, which uses half of the worldwide consumption of PBDEs. According to studies conducted in Europe and the US, a small dose of PBDEs fed to newborn laboratory mice and rats disrupts brain development, alters learning ability, memory function, behaviour and hearing. Mice fed less than 1 part per million of PBDEs performed poorly in maze tests, were hyperactive and slower to adjust to new situations.

NOTE: Some Chapters commence with what I call *instant information for busy parents*. This concisely sums up the particular Chapter.

PART ONE

Causes of the problems

CHAPTER ONE

Politics and causes

Instant information for busy parents

While there are several known causes of ASD, the most serious and universal (and 'stoppable') are reactions to various aspects of immunisation.

You will not be told about the full extent of these by Government Immunisation agencies. Even the many deaths are kept quiet. (For a full explanation of these facts, see books such as *Vaccination – the Right Choice* by para-legal expert Maureen Hickman or see the Australian Vaccination Network website (www.avn.org.au) or Vaccine Information Service (www.vaccination.inoz.com)

Other known behavioural problem causes include antibiotic overuse resulting in gut problems affecting the brain; heavy metals, like lead, arsenic and mercury (supplied to children free-of-charge in some vaccines) affect behaviour, learning, neuron damage and the immune system; common chemicals, food dyes, and reactions to some foods cause further autoimmune reactions in some ASD children; birthing problems affect a small percentage.

These are all dealt with in detail in this book, plus their politics in this Chapter.

Multiple ADHD/Autism spectrum disease class-actions are now taking place around the world. They are occurring in nations whose Governments cause their citizens to closely follow the American model of immunisation. In the UK thousands of families are ready to commence actions following six test cases that commenced in 2003. Lawsuits began in the USA in 2001, where in many States the filed actions are asking for a jury trial of all pharmaceutical companies involved in the production of vaccines containing mercury.

Mercury poisoning from vaccines: a generation at risk

A full generation of children in America (and similar in the United Kingdom and Australia) was exposed to dangerous doses of highly toxic ethyl mercury from 1990 through 2000. Children were injected with the toxic mercury that was a major ingredient in a chemical product called thimerosal, an additive and biological preservative packaged into multi-dose vials of many childhood vaccines. With each dose of vaccine that contained thimerosal, a child would also get an injection of toxic mercury. Each one of those mercury injections exposed the child to levels of toxic mercury in excess of the federal government's own safety guidelines.

Mercury is widely known to cause neurological damage, often permanent. Current clinical and epidemiological research suggests that the mercury-laden thimerosal so widely given to children by the drug companies in the 1990's might cause a range of neurological and neurodevelopmental injuries, including ADHD and autism. Compounding this public health disaster is that the toxic exposure was entirely avoidable. The thimerosal was added merely as product packaging for the multi-dose vials, and is not needed as a preservative when the vaccines are packaged in single-dose vials or single-use syringes. Thimerosal had nothing to do with vaccine safety, and everything to do with the profits and convenience of packaging for the pharmaceutical companies.

Government and drug company response

The US federal government recommended in 1999 that the drug companies should provide a thimerosal-free vaccine supply by the summer of 2001, but allowed the continued use of vaccine products containing thimerosal. On October 1, 2001, the Institute of Medicine (IOM) went one step further, urging that all remaining stocks of thimerosal-laced vaccines be removed from use immediately and destroyed. Amazingly, the drug companies refused to tell the IOM how much mercury-laced vaccine product remained on the market and in use. The IOM also called for extensive and immediate scientific and clinical studies to assess this critical health issue, but could not identify where the money for this needed research will come from.

Why functional methods are not in general medical use

Big money is made by 'hooking' a child for much of his early life on some pharmaceutical psyche drug (sometimes not even approved for children). As you will read in Chapter Five, fairly simple methods bring amazing changes without drugs. Therefore the child is not 'hooked' on anything. That is bad for business. If you think this is a radical statement, think again. This true story tells a thousand words:

The Director of an Australian Vaccination Information Network told me how a letter was sent to the then current Federal Government Department of Health. The letter proposed a simple study that would cost very little to perform, using available statistics. This would compare the health of vaccinated children with the health of unvaccinated children. A Government Minister replied personally. This is an outline of what he said, *"**We will not do this study because you may find the unvaccinated children healthier. If that was found then it would change our Government's policy. We would not do that.**"*

What he meant was this – our 'health' policy has little to do with your child's health.

It is very necessary for you to understand that you cannot always trust what Government and media medical 'experts' tell us.[70] A good illustration occurred in Australia in the late 1990's when the Minister for Health Dr Wooldridge announced[71] that, *"It is more likely for a child to be killed by a meteorite than die from immunization."*

This was plainly different to the facts, as in the previous 21 months, seven children had been reported to the Canberra-based Adverse Reactions Unit to have died following immunisation. If even one child anywhere in the world had been hit and killed by a meteorite the matter would have been headline news. Vaccine deaths decidedly do not 'hit' the headlines. Most of our media is, in effect, controlled by their unquestioning belief in 'experts'.

What we are **not** told is often more important than what we **are** told. For instance, the Government Immunisation website tells us that immunisation is 'safe and effective'. Neither of these is true. For something to be safe it must be safe for everyone. If a toy is found to be possibly unsafe it is taken off the market. The very presence and need of the Government's own Vaccine Adverse Reactions Events Unit tells us vaccines are not safe for everyone. There is no Adverse Events unit for toys. One 'adverse event' and bingo! it's off the market. Not so with vaccines. As just stated, deaths have been admitted to be directly related to vaccines by this Unit. Not one, but many. What would happen to a toy that killed several children? The maker would face Court.

What about 'effective'? For something to be 'effective' usually means a minimum 95% effectiveness. If you buy a new car you expect 100% effectiveness, everything working. But there are maybe 5% of new cars that have problems. Vaccines are far less effective than 95% – some maybe only 40%. What is 'effective' anyway? If time is taken into account, then many vaccines effectiveness is NIL beyond a certain number of years. Worse, evidence is mounting that mothers no longer pass natural immunity on to their children – because of their own immunization they themselves never gained natural immunity. This has many implications. Possibly chief among these is the spate of babies dying without apparent reason (labelled SIDS) and the parents blamed and often gaoled. If the unthinkable happens and more than one child in a family dies in this way, the parents may face murder charges. Fortunately, in recent years pathology has discovered familial genetic weakness can cause a defective immune system. This genetic weakness, it is believed, can be caused by childhood immunisation. A mother may simply be unable to pass on essential immune system information. This can result in an uncontrolled spread of certain pathogens (enemy bacteria) in a child, at times leading to death. Such incidences are more frequent than ever before. It is believed that immunisation, which does not produce a normal immunity, can rob a woman of the ability to pass on a complete immune message to the newborn. This could eventuallly lead to total dependence on vaccine companies for protection that a healthy immune system gives naturally.

Because of immunization problems in Japan, including cases of meningitis, the Government there banned MMR Vaccine in 1993.

The following is a report by US writer and medical osteopath Dr Joeseph Mercola, a 'whistle-blower' and editor of the world's third most read medical website (www.mercola.com).

> "Japan is virtually the only developed nation to turn its back on the vaccine. Government health chiefs claim a four-year experiment with it has had serious financial and human costs.
>
> Of the 3,969 medical compensation claims relating to vaccines in the last 30 years, a quarter had been made by those badly affected by the combined measles, mumps and rubella vaccine, they say.
>
> The MMR was banned in Japan in 1993 after 1.8 million children had been given two types of MMR and a record number developed non-viral meningitis and other adverse reactions were recorded.
>
> Official figures show there were three deaths while eight children were left with permanent handicaps ranging from damaged hearing and blindness to loss of control of limbs.
>
> The government reconsidered using MMR in 1999 but decided it was safer to keep the ban and continue using individual vaccines for measles, mumps and rubella.
>
> The British Department of Health said Japan had used a type of MMR, which included a strain of mumps vaccine that had particular problems and was discontinued in the UK because of safety concerns.
>
> The Japanese government realized there was a problem with MMR soon after its introduction in April 1989 when vaccination

was compulsory. Parents who refused had to pay a small fine.

An analysis of vaccinations over a three-month period showed one in every 900 children was experiencing problems.

This was over 2,000 times higher than the expected rate of one child in every 100,000 to 200,000.

The health ministry switched to another MMR vaccine in October 1991 but the incidence was still high with one in 1,755 children affected. No separate record has been kept of claims involving autism.

Tests on the spinal fluid of 125 children affected were carried out to see if the vaccine had got into the children's nervous systems. They found one confirmed case and two further suspected cases. In 1993, after a public outcry fuelled by worries over the flu vaccine, the government dropped the requirement for children to be vaccinated against measles or rubella.

Dr Hiroki Nakatani, director of the Infectious Disease Division at Japan's Ministry of Health and Welfare said that giving individual vaccines cost twice as much as MMR 'but we believe it is worth it'."

For the information in this short pre-Chapter introduction, I am also indebted to the non-profit organisation Centre for Media and Democracy (USA) investigative journalists, John Stauber and Sheldon Rampton whose books[17] are now being widely read throughout the world. They are successfully unmasking unusual professional and business conduct in the medical and general media. When children's health is at risk, that maybe a very serious mistake. Parents are naturally protective, much like a lioness is of her cubs. Once the enemy is identified, it is best to be somewhere else.

Their latest book *Trust Us – We're Experts,* should be required reading for every parent. They point out that pharmaceutical ads in medical journals are often deceiving. One team of medical investigators suggested that doctors use caution when reviewing such ads. One biostatistician was paid $10,000 for writing a single eight paragraph letter published in the *Journal of the American Medical Association.*

The British medical journal *The Lancet* published a study of 100 promotional claims for blood pressure and cholesterol-lowering drugs in medical journals with references to research that did not support the advertisements' claims 44 percent of the time.

For blood pressure medications, references were misleading some 69 percent of the time. Most commonly, references were found to be **"particularly misleading"**. (*Lancet January 4, 2003; 361)*

Dr Mercola commented:

> "Through September of last year (2001) the FDA has told companies to fix distorted ads just 18 times. This is off the pace from last year when 64 warnings were issued for the full year. Drug companies spent more than $19 billion last year to promote their products to consumers and doctors. That is nearly double the amount that was spent four years ago. This is also one of the major contributing factors as to *why physicians are the third leading cause of death.*
>
> In the US, physicians rely on drugs to patch up the problem, rather than seeking the cause."

In 2002, thirteen editors of the western world's leading medical journals[18] wrote a joint statement complaining to the drug companies of their unethical practices. These practices often included writing their own research article for publication and then paying a well-known professor or leading clinician in the particular field to put his name to it. For instance, sometimes as much as $30,000 was paid to a cancer authority, who thus sold his name to promote methods that may or may not be effective or even safe.

Not all okay drugs are okay – some are approved to kill

The New York Times No.1 best selling book *The People's Pharmacy* (Joe Graedon & Terresa Graedon PH.D) tells us that, "Safety is a relative concept. People assume that when the FDA gives its seal of approval, a new drug is safe and effective. Wrong, WRONG, **wrong!** We said it in the first edition and repeat with more emphasis today – there is no such thing as a safe drug."

The authors quote an internal FDA memo from Dr Paul Leber (then Director of the FDA's Division of Neuropharmacological Drugs to Dr Robert Temple (then director of the FDA's Office of Drug Evaluation). The memo concerns the migraine drug 'Imitrex' (sumatriptan), which was released by SmithKline Beecham in 1993.

> "Used appropriately, Imitrex is reasonably safe; if used in a patient with pre-existing cardiovascular disease, however, it may be dangerous, even deadly ... The Division's recommendation to approve the Imitrex NDA (New Drug Application) reflects a risk assessment which, in common with all such determinations, turns as much on personal values and implicitly held private assumptions as it does on evidence and reassign.

In sum, a case can be made that, from a viewpoint of public health, the benefit accruing to the population of migraineurs is outweighed by the injury and fatalities that Imitrex's marketing seems certain to cause."

This drug appears to have killed an unknown number of users around the world. Because of the litigations now being sought, the present manufacturer Glaxo has recently changed the package insert to warn that deaths attributed to cardiovascular events or strokes have occurred within hours of taking sumatriptan.

The authors of *The People's Pharmacy* point out that, "The really shocking story is that everybody but the consumer understands this dangerous game ... One does not have to be a pharmacologist to see that the FDA is playing Russian roulette with us."

Congressional investigators have pointed out that lives could have been saved if the FDA monitored drugs and vaccines more carefully after marketing, and reported complications to physicians and parents. Say the authors, "But to this day [1998] the agency falls short on several counts. It has no organised, scientific method of tracking adverse drug reactions and interactions. When problems are uncovered, there is no efficient way to alert people to dangers or controversies ... It's a pharmacy free-for-all."

These lessons also apply to vaccines. Possibly even more so, as proper tests for vaccines have never been carried out. Package inserts say that no testing for cancer or mutagenic events has been done. Since several of the many ingredients that make up a typical vaccine are known to cause auto-immune responses, and some have been known to cause cancer (simian virus) – maybe this is the reason why so many doctors and paediatricians have refused to be vaccinated themselves[19].

(Since the 1997 edition of *The People's Pharmacy*, some steps have been taken to mend these matters, particularly in regard to drug interactions. In Australia, the job of warning customers was primarily taken on by caring members of the Pharmacy Guild who initiated useful computer based print-outs for customers.)

Summary

From the cover of *Trust Us – We're Experts:*[22] "We count on the experts ... We should stop trusting them right this second."

This book question everything that concerns your health or the health of your children. In Australia the law demands full disclosure of all 'material risks' in medical procedures.[23] Do not blindly trust what you hear in medical announcements via the media. For instance, contrary to media reporting, smallpox vaccinations are in fact ***not*** harmless according to medical research. Nor is Hepatitis B vaccination 'safe and necessary for all children'. You will read the truth later in this book.

An article by a well-known American medical writer, Marc K Siegel illustrates "why parents have become suspicious of the information promulgated about vaccine safety by so called medical 'experts'. Dr Siegel states that 'A temporary ban on the measles vaccine in England in the late 90s led to the deaths of several children from measles'. Fact is, there has never been a ban, temporary or otherwise, on measles vaccine in England, and certainly not in the 1990s. No child has died of measles in England for over 20 years or more. Dr Siegel's research appears to be sloppy in the extreme."

Bill Walsh, Chairman, *Action against Autism*, Scotland, UK

This was an unusual mistake for Dr Siegel who normally writes well-informed pieces in the *Los Angeles Times*, the *New York Times* and other publications.

CHAPTER TWO

Behind the scenes

The carefully hidden political/financial/medical battle behind the scenes that mask major true reasons for our children's world-wide ASD epidemic.

Many serious adverse reactions are linked to vaccines authorised and recommended by the US Centers for Disease Control and Prevention (CDC). The CDC controls the listing of vaccinations that doctors inject into children, effectively worldwide. They also supposedly monitor vaccine safety by keeping track of possible side effects. The number of recommended vaccines for children has doubled since the late1980s. It is now reported that evidence is indicating the CDC has a cosy relationship to vaccine manufacturers.[82] For instance, the CDC's Vaccine Advisory Committee is paid money by vaccine manufacturers. Other close ties include sharing a vaccine patent, owning stock in a vaccine company, obtaining public money to monitor manufacturer vaccine tests and other payments for research.

One media agency reported, **"Critics say the organization, which says its goal is to protect the public from disease and vaccine side effects, represents a conflict of interest that could hurt or kill people and children."** (*United Press International*, July 21, 2003)

"We are in the midst of an international epidemic. Those responsible for investigating and dealing with this epidemic have failed", according to Dr Andrew Wakefield[32] (British pediatric gastroenterologist, discoverer of the gut-brain connection in MMR vaccination).

This revealing and daring public declaration was made before a gathering at the Washington Rally on Capitol Hill, Washington DC in April 2002. The epidemic he described was of autism spectrum disorders, now affecting six in every one hundred children in USA[33], and UK and fast approaching those numbers in Australia. Dr Wakefield's medical work was later endorsed by an Editorial in the prestigious *American Journal of Gastroenterology* (September 2000: Volume 95, see text in endnote 32 ibid.).

The rally was organised by a federation of American ASD Associations, representing some 3½ million children and young people affected by one or more of the learning/behavourial problems related to ASD. The epidemic is highlighted by the United States Department of Education statistics for autism since 1991 (5,400 autistic students) compared to 2001 (79,000).

This includes a sharp (25% rise annually) from 1997 to 2001 (totalling 45,000). **Now, in 2003, the rise has become even steeper, illustrated by the *daily* new cases in California (pop. 34 million) rising from 5 (1991) daily to 84 weekly (2003).** Similar rises have been recorded around the western world. In Australia (pop. 19 million), 17 new cases are now presenting weekly, and rising.

These figures are a terrible increase on the two in ten thousand children with autism prior to the 1980's.

To these totals must be added the numerous numbers of other autism spectrum disorders (Aspergers, Tourette's, and Retts syndrome and many children with borderline autistic-like symptoms and learning problems, such as ODD, ADHD, ADD, etc).

Until recently, these figures were disputed by the Establishment who claimed 'better diagnosis' (autism is hard NOT to diagnose!), 'population migration' (all States have similar rises), or 'new criteria' (strict criteria began in 1996) caused an 'apparent' rise (trying to place these children, the US Dept. Education found it all too real, and State aid even more so). However, in 2003, studies by the Centres for Disease Control admitted a true and alarming rise. For political, legal and financial reasons, the causes are still disputed. Dr Wakefield was the pioneer who found evidence of vaccine induced autism. For this he was forced to resign from his post at the Royal Free Hospital in London.

Dr Wakefield's 'crime' was alerting the medical world to the findings of his team working with autistic children after a massive MMR vaccination program in England (1995).[34] His Royal Free Hospital group were the first to find evidence of a connection between gut damage, measles virus, autism and vaccines. Several of the families in his first 50 cases had seen immediate changes in their children post-vaccination.

He eventually resigned under duress from the hospital and his work obfuscated and denied. Today, Wakefield works at a multi-million dollar American Foundation that has confirmed his own discoveries, now replicated by world-wide research – but still opposed using 'shonky' facts by the vested interests.[35,36] None of the industry or Government studies opposing his work actually studied the children or questioned the parents. They were based on what are called 'epidemiological' studies, the interpretation of mass statistics. More alarming still, Centres for Disease Control scientists re-wrote a study document on a link between the ASD's and a preservative used in many multivalent vaccines (more than one vaccine per shot, eg MMR) called thimerosal, which contain 50% of the neurologically toxic metal, ethyl mercury. As children have multiple vaccinations and mercury is cumulative, American, British and Australian children received up to 100 times the 'allowed' mercury intake.[37] This mercury load is now found to be one of the factors in vaccines that cause ASD's.[38]

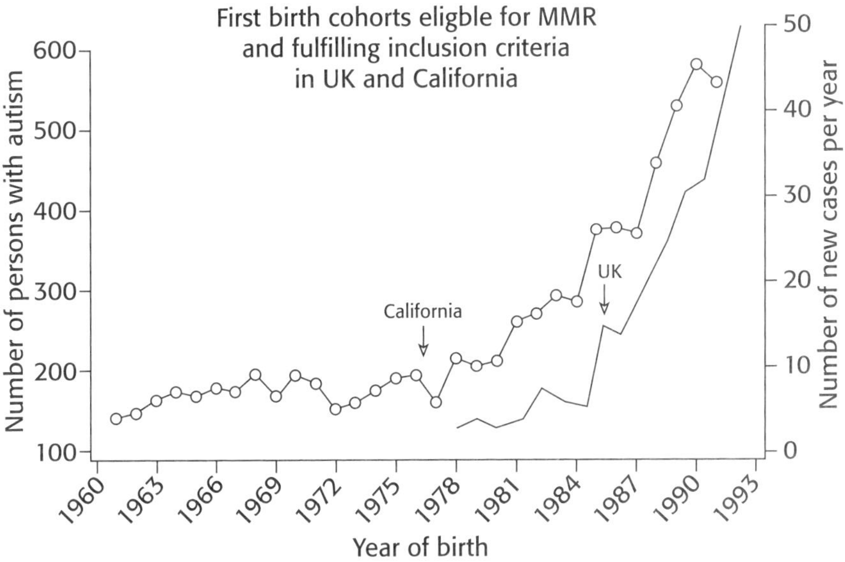

In February 1998, Andrew Wakefield published results of a small study, in which he described, for the first time, some specific changes in the ileum (small intestine) and colon of children with autism and suggested a possible relationship with the measles-mumps-rubella (MMR) vaccination. This and subsequent publications by the same team have changed the way parents perceive autism and vaccination. The attack on Wakefield and his work by the vaccine authorities and the pro-vaccine lobby was prompt, massive and relentless. Part of this was dissemination of propaganda.

Establishment quotes flawed studies ignores new work

Two publications by a team from Finland are most often quoted. In both, the authors describe the adverse events reported following the administration of some 3 million doses of MMR vaccine to about 1.8 million individuals during a national immunization campaign in Finland between 1982 and 1996. The main authors of the two publications in question were H. Peltola and A. Patja and both stated that there was no evidence for MMR vaccine-associated inflammatory bowel disease or autism in the 14-year study.

But many experts have criticized the study findings and its conclusions because:

1 fewer than 200 individuals (those who had developed acute events **within only 3 weeks of vaccination)** were followed for 14 years. The rest of the 1.8 million vaccine-recipients were not.
2 **Both regressive autism and inflammatory bowel disease (IBD) are chronic illnesses, which develop over months or years. No one ever claimed that they start within 21 days of vaccination.**
3 Wakefield never contended that children who develop diarrhoea immediately after vaccination, a known and accepted reaction, are those who will go on to develop IBD as young adults.
4 The Finnish study ended in 1996. Autism and IBD were never mentioned in connection with MMR vaccination prior to 1998
5 **Peltola stated on BBC Radio-4 on January 13, 2001 that the study was not designed to look at IBD and autism**
6 The vaccine manufacturer funded the study.

Thanks to an expensive and extensive media campaign, the pro-vaccine lobby prevailed with the media. The study findings are constantly interpreted in the press, and over the Internet, as proving that there was no increase in autism and IBD in the millions who received the MMR vaccine during the vaccination campaign in Finland and were followed for 14 years. Obviously, this is not true as there has been a significant rise in autism and inflammatory bowel disease in Finland in recent years.[39]

> *Wikinews*, January 18, 2005
>
> Stockholm – A well-known Swedish doctor and researcher at Gothenburg University has been prosecuted, together with the Vice-Chancellor and the President of the University Coucil, for failing to hand over sensitive data on patients to outside critics.
>
> The Parliamentary Ombudsman, an official appointed by the Parliament, decide to press charges against professor Christopher Gillberg md, professor Gunnar Svedberg (Vice-Chancellor) and Arne Wittlöv (President), for failing to comply with a court order from February 2003.

Now, four years later, the truth or 'untruth' of these widely used media claims that there is no connection between mercury in vaccines and ASD problems has been revealed. Professor Gillberg has been prosecuted for refusing to hand over evidence that would disprove these claims.[84]

M. Kielinen et al, in a study published in the *Journal of European Child & Adolescent Psychiatry* described a significant rise in autism in the northern provinces of Finland. The Kielinen study included all children born in the two provinces, between 1979 and 1994. Every single one of those children was eligible and must have received the MMR vaccine. The authors personally reviewed all records of children with autism to determine that they fulfilled the criteria. The cumulative incidence of autism was 12.2/10,000, a significant increase when compared to the previously reported incidence of 4.75/10,000 by Vinni and Timonen (1991). The increase in the younger children, all born in the second half of the MMR campaign, was even more striking. In the 5 to 7 age group, the cumulative incidence was 20.7/10,000 or more than 1 in 500. Aspergers is now four times this rate (Yazbak, 2002).

"There is no reason to doubt that this increase is not occurring nationwide nor that it is less spectacular than in other European countries." (Commentary by Dr Edward Yazbak FAAP, pediatrician and researcher, Mass. USA.)

Conflicts of interest that affect Australians

The US Federal Congress has become involved in this controversy both for health reasons and for possible conflicts of interest between the approval process for these vaccines and the pharmaceutical industry. In fact, this conflict of interest has led to several Congressional hearings which commenced in 2001 and continued into 2003. The resulting Congressional report found that the pharmaceutical industry exerted undue influence on mandatory vaccine legislation. The report stated that, "The vaccine approval process has also been contaminated by flawed or incomplete clinical trials, and government officials have chosen to ignore negative results."

In response, Congressman Dan Burton (R-Indiana) and others called for the removal of all vaccines containing thimerosal. They have called on the government to insist on using available vaccines that do not contain thimerosal.

Then in May 2003 came this landmark declaration from the US Congress Committee investigating the alarming increase in ASD:

Mercury in medicine – taking unnecessary risks

A report prepared by the staff of the Subcommittee on Human Rights and Wellness Committee on Government Reform, United States House of Representatives, Chairman Dan Burton, May 2003. (This report is the result of a 3-year investigation initiated by the Committee on Government Reform.)

I. Executive Summary

Vaccines are the only medicines that American citizens are mandated to receive as a condition for school and day care attendance, and in some instances, employment. Additionally, families who receive federal assistance are also required to show proof that their children have been fully immunized. While the mandate for which vaccines must be administered is a state mandate, it is the Federal Government, through the Centres for Disease Control and Prevention (CDC) and its Advisory Committee for Immunization Practices that make the Universal Immunization Recommendations to which the majority of states defer when determining mandates. Since the early to mid-1990's, Congress has been concerned about the danger posed by mercury in medical applications, and in 1997, directed the Food and Drug Administration (FDA) to evaluate the human exposure to mercury through foods and drugs.

In 1999, following up on the FDA evaluation and pursuant to its authority, the House Committee on Government Reform initiated an investigation into the dangers of exposure to mercury through vaccination. The investigation later expanded to examine the potential danger posed through exposure to mercury in dental amalgams.[40] This full committee investigation complemented and built upon the investigations initiated by two of its subcommittees. In January 2003, the investigation continued in the newly formed Subcommittee on Human Rights and Wellness.

A primary concern that arose early in the investigation of vaccine safety was the exposure of infants and young children to mercury, a known toxin, through mandatory childhood immunizations. This concern had been raised as a possible underlying factor in the dramatic rise in rates of late-onset or 'acquired' autism. The symptoms of autism are markedly similar to those of mercury poisoning. Significant concern has been raised about the continued use of mercury in medical applications decades after the recognition that mercury can be harmful, especially to our most vulnerable population – our children. This report will address one form of mercury in medical applications, thimerosal, as a preservative in vaccines.

In July 2000, it was estimated that 8,000 children a day were being exposed to mercury in excess of Federal guidelines through their mandatory vaccines.

One leading researcher made the following statement to the Committee in July 2000, "There's no question that mercury does not belong in vaccines. There are other compounds that could be used as preservatives. And everything we know about childhood susceptibility, neurotoxicity of mercury at the foetus and at the infant level, points out that we should not have these fetuses and infants exposed to mercury. There's no need of it in the vaccines."

The Food and Drug Administration's (FDA) mission is to "promote and protect the public health by helping safe and effective products reach the market in a timely way, and monitoring products for continued safety after they are in use." However, the FDA uses a subjective barometer in determining when a product that has known risks can remain on the market. According to the agency, "at the heart of all FDA's product evaluation decisions is a judgment about whether a new product's benefits to users will outweigh its risks. No regulated product is totally risk-free, so these judgments are important. FDA will allow a product to present more of a risk when its potential benefit is great – especially for products used to treat serious, life-threatening conditions."

This argument – that the known risks of infectious diseases outweigh a potential risk of neurological damage from exposure to thimerosal in vaccines, is one that has continuously been presented to the Committee by government officials. FDA officials have stressed that any possible risk from thimerosal was theoretical: that no proof of harm existed. Upon a thorough review of the scientific literature and internal documents from government and industry, the Committee did in fact find evidence that thimerosal posed a risk. The possible risk for harm from either low dose chronic or one time high level (bolus dose) exposure to thimerosal is not 'theoretical', but very real and documented in the medical literature.

Congress has long been concerned about the human exposure to mercury through medical applications. As a result of these concerns, in 1997, Congress instructed the FDA to evaluate the human exposure to mercury through drugs and foods. Through this Congressionally mandated evaluation, the FDA realized that the amount of ethyl mercury infants were exposed to in the first six months of life through their mandatory vaccinations exceeded the Environmental Protection Agency's (EPA) limit for a closely associated compound methyl mercury. The FDA and other Federal agencies determined that in the absence of a specific standard for ethylmercury, the limits for ingested methyl mercury should be used for injected ethyl mercury. The Institute of Medicine, in 2000, evaluated the EPA's methyl mercury standard and determined that based upon scientific data that it, rather than the FDA's, was the scientifically validated safe exposure standard.

Rather than acting aggressively to remove thimerosal from children's vaccines, the FDA and other agencies within the Department of Health and Human Services (HHS) adopted an incremental approach that allowed children to continue to be exposed to ethyl mercury from vaccines for more than two additional years. In fact, in 2001, the Centres for Disease Control and Prevention (CDC) refused even to express a preference for thimerosal-free vaccines, despite the fact that thimerosal had been removed from almost every childhood vaccine produced for use in the United States.

On three occasions in the last 15 years, changes have been made to vaccine policies to reduce the risk of serious adverse effects. First, a transition from oral polio vaccine to injected polio was accomplished in the United States to reduce the transmission of vaccine-induced polio. Second, an acellular pertussis vaccine was developed and a transition from DTP to DTaP was accomplished to reduce the risk of pertussis – induced seizures in children. And third, when the Rotashield vaccine for rotavirus was linked to a serious bowel condition (intersucception), it was removed from the US market. Ethyl mercury has been largely removed from every major childhood vaccine manufactured for use in the United States, except the influenza vaccine, which continues to contain trace amounts.

This success, however, does not change the fact that millions of American children were exposed to levels of mercury through vaccines that exceeded comparable federal guidelines. Many parents, and a growing number of scientists, believe that this mercury exposure may have contributed to the explosive growth in autism spectrum disorders, and neurological and behavioural disorders that this country has experienced. The scientific evidence in this area is considered by some to still be inconclusive, in large part due to the lack of serious, effective inquiry by our health agencies. The federal government has an obligation to vigorously pursue the necessary research to determine the extent of the impact of these heightened exposures to ethyl mercury on our population.

A second concern that arose during the investigation was the continued use of mercury in dental amalgams. Mercury has been used as a component in dental fillings since the Civil War era. The American Dental Association and its member dentists have taken a position that the mercury in fillings, which are considered toxic until placed in the tooth, and is considered toxic when removed from the mouth, is completely safe while in the human mouth. This position seems counter even to the ADA-funded research that shows the daily release of small amounts of mercury vapours in the human mouth where dental amalgams are present, as well as minute chipping and swallowing of the mercury fillings over time.

Babies and young children are exposed to this additional mercury. As developing foetuses, babies are exposed to mercury through the placenta. If pregnant women have mercury amalgams, they are unknowingly excreting low levels of mercury on a daily basis to their foetuses. Additionally, children who receive dental services through Medicaid are also potentially exposed to mercury. When these children need dental fillings, because of the low cost, only mercury amalgams are available for use. This concern remains under investigation by the Subcommittee on Human Rights and Wellness.

II. Findings

Through this investigation of paediatric vaccine safety, the following findings are made:

1. Mercury is hazardous to humans. Its use in medicinal products is undesirable, unnecessary and should be minimized or eliminated entirely.
2. For decades, ethyl mercury was used extensively in medical products ranging from vaccines to topical ointments as preservative and an anti-bacteriological agent.
3. Manufacturers of vaccines and thimerosal, (an ethyl mercury compound used in vaccines), have never conducted adequate testing on the safety of thimerosal. The FDA has never required manufacturers to conduct adequate safety testing on thimerosal and ethyl mercury compounds.
4. Studies and papers documenting the hypoallergenicity and toxicity of thimerosal (ethyl mercury) have existed for decades.
5. Autism in the United States has grown at epidemic proportions during the last decade. By some estimates the number of autistic children in the United States is growing between 10 and 17 percent per year. The medical community has been unable to determine the underlying cause(s) of this explosive growth.
6. At the same time that the incidence of autism was growing, the number of childhood vaccines containing thimerosal was growing, increasing the amount of ethyl mercury to which infants were exposed threefold.
7. A growing number of scientists and researchers believe that a relationship between the increase in neurodevelopmental disorders of autism, attention deficit hyperactive disorder, and speech or language delay, and the increased use of thimerosal in vaccines is plausible and deserves more scrutiny. In 2001, the

Institute of Medicine determined that such a relationship is biologically plausible, but that not enough evidence exists to support or reject this hypothesis.

8 The FDA acted too slowly to remove ethyl mercury from over-the-counter products like topical ointments and skin creams. Although an advisory committee determined that ethyl mercury was unsafe in these products in 1980, a rule requiring its removal was not finalized until 1998.

9 The FDA and the CDC failed in their duty to be vigilant as new vaccines containing thimerosal were approved and added to the immunization schedule. When the Hepatitis B and Haemophilus Influenzae Type B vaccines were added to the recommended schedule of childhood immunizations, the cumulative amount of ethyl mercury to which children were exposed nearly tripled.

10 The amount of ethyl mercury to which children were exposed through vaccines prior to the 1999 announcement exceeded two safety thresholds established by the Federal government for a closely related substance-methyl mercury. While the Federal Government has established no safety threshold for ethyl mercury, experts agree that the methyl mercury guidelines are a good substitute. Federal health officials have conceded that the amount of thimerosal in vaccines exceeded the EPA threshold of 0.1 micrograms per kilogram of bodyweight. In fact, the amount of mercury in one dose of DTaP or Hepatitis B vaccines (25 micrograms each) exceeded this threshold many times over. Federal health officials have not conceded that this amount of thimerosal in vaccines exceeded the FDA's more relaxed threshold of 0.4 micrograms per kilogram of body weight. In most cases, however, it clearly did.

11 The actions taken by the HHS to remove thimerosal from vaccines in 1999 were not sufficiently aggressive. As a result, thimerosal remained in some vaccines for an additional two years.

12 The CDC's failure to state a preference for thimerosal-free vaccines in 2000 and 2001 was an abdication of their responsibility. As a result, many children received vaccines containing thimerosal when thimerosal-free alternatives were available.

13 The Influenza vaccine appears to be the sole remaining vaccine given to children in the United States on a regular basis that contains thimerosal. Two formulations recommended for children six months of age or older continue to contain trace amounts of thimerosal. Thimerosal should be removed from these vaccines. No amount of mercury is appropriate in any childhood vaccine.

14 The CDC in general and the National Immunization Program in particular are conflicted in their duties to monitor the safety of vaccines, while also charged with the responsibility of purchasing vaccines for resale and promoting increased immunization rates.

15 There is inadequate research regarding ethyl mercury neurotoxicity (damage to nerves) and nephrotoxicity (kidney damage).

16 There is inadequate research regarding the relationship between autism and the use of mercury-containing vaccines.

17 To date, studies conducted or funded by the CDC that purportedly dispute any correlation between autism and vaccine injury have been of poor design, under-powered, and fatally flawed. The CDC's rush to support and promote such research is reflective of a philosophical conflict in looking fairly at emerging theories and clinical data related to adverse reactions from vaccinations.

Summary of science review that influenced Congress

> *"The characteristics of autism and mercury poisoning, derived from a review of medical literature, have been found, upon comparison, to be strikingly similar. The parallels between the two diseases are so close that it would be unreasonable to assume that the similarities occur by chance. The exposure route is childhood vaccines, most of which contain thimerosal, a preservative comprised of 50% ethyl mercury by weight. The amount of mercury a typical child under two years receives from vaccinations equates to 237.5 micrograms".*[41]

Testimony before Congress 2002
Sallie Bernard, Albert Enayati, B.S., Ch.E., M.S.M.E. Heidi Roger, Teresa Binstock, Lyn Redwood, R.N., M.S.N., C.R.N.P., Woody McGinnis, M.D.

Massive class-actions – the greatest consumer scandal in history?

See also Appendix III

By 2001, because of the evidence now emerging against both the US Government agencies and vaccine manufacturers, 1500 class actions had been launched by parents with ASD children. Nearly all of these had seen their child regress after various vaccinations. Some had seen their child die. A spokesman from one of the law firms said that "if our cases are found correct, then this will be the greatest consumer scandal in history." [42]

The same commences in the UK in February, 2004, with 1500 parents in class-actions. When will they begin in Australia?

While parents were struggling to make hard decisions involving the safety of their *children* with vaccination, they receive mixed messages from the experts. Though no vaccines are perfectly safe the FDA had gone from deeming thimerosal unsafe to asking vaccine manufacturers to voluntarily phase-out thimerosal from their products. People wondered if the vaccines containing thimerosal were in fact safe to use while clinics were using up the extra supplies they had kept stock of since the 1998 FDA request.

Vaccination may *damage* children in several ways (see Appendix III, 'Journey into the land of make believe'). Live or attenuated virus vaccination can actually produce the infection that the vaccine is supposed to prevent. For example, live polio should never be administered to a child who comes in contact with an HIV patient, for the attenuated virus can 'leap' to the HIV patient and produce polio. Reports exist of normal parents who have developed polio from the viral vaccine given to their children.

A second mechanism of damage comes from *neurotoxic materials* found sometimes in vaccines. thimerosal is the most widely discussed, since it contains mercury. The amount is small. Each vaccine is equivalent to the amount of mercury found in a 200g/6oz can of tuna fish. Nevertheless, some argue that even these levels may be important in a vulnerable child.

The third, and probably the most important theory of vaccine damage, relates to allergic reactions and the development of an auto-immune response, stimulated by the vaccine and its adjuvant (see Chapter Two). Vaccines always contain adjuvants, which are substances known to amplify the body's response to the vaccine. These adjuvants are known to sometimes cause allergic and auto-immune responses on their own. [43,44]

Disclosure of risks is obligatory

None of this is told to parents. There is no balanced advice given. This is contrary to a major precedent Supreme Court case in Australia (Rogers vs Whitaker, 1992), where the judgement was given that all material risks must be given in regards to any medical procedure.

(Mercury was supposed to have ceased to be used in Australia, at least in MMR vaccines, approximately August 2002. As at Feb 2003, Hg is still used in Hep B childhood vaccine (<1 umg), and most flu vaccines (50 umg).

Vaccination not compulsory in Australia

If you wish to avoid vaccination and build-up your child's immune system instead see Chapters 8 through to 20. Contrary to popular belief (the result of heavy propaganda), vaccination in Australia not compulsory.

Maternity Immunisation Allowance (MIA)

This Australian federal government allowance is paid after 18 months of age, when the baby is either fully immunised **or is exempt from immunisation**. MIA is paid in addition to Maternity Allowance.

Exemptions?

To receive these benefits without being fully immunised your immunisation provider needs to certify that:

- Your child has a medical reason not to have a particular vaccination;
- Your child has had a disease and has aquired natural immunity;
- A particular vaccine is unavailable; or
- ***You have made a formal conscientious objection because of personal, philosophical, religious or medical beliefs to your child being immunised.***

You will need to ask your immunisation provider to sign a 'Conscientious Objection' form.

Vaccine injuries

If your child is vaccine injured contact your national non-government consumer vaccination network for a list of law firms that specialise in cases of this nature.

In Australia, these are some of the law firms that specialise.

Queensland
Grays Lawyers
07 3846 2286

Victoria
Maurice Blackburn & Co
03 9345 2768

Western Australia
Fordhams (Subiaco)
08 9388 8899

New South Wales
Carters Law Firm
02 9649 0233

South Australia
Corsers
08 8223 6788

PART II

Reversing the problems

CHAPTER THREE

What happens in our child's body?

Instant information for parents with little time

If they reach the brain, some foods – especially those containing peptides (protein particles) of gluten (bread and grains) and casein (milk and cheese) – are now well-known to cause ADHD /autism-type symptoms, learning problems and sometimes hyperactivity. According to statistics gathered over 36 years by the American Autism Research Institute from 22,300 parent reports, removing these foods caused immediate improvements to take place in a high percentage of these children.[45] Upon removing milk and all dairy from the diet, 48% got better. Upon removing milk and gluten, 64% got better. Just removing chocolate caused 49% of ASD children to improve. I constantly see these same results among my own clients.

Gluten is found in most grains (except rice, buckwheat, millet and corn) and casein in mammalian milk of all kinds (i.e. not in soy or rice milk). As you will read in a later Chapter, they are both opioids, or morphine-like substances under certain circumstances. To reach the brain they must first be able to get through a barrier in the gut wall that will normally only allow 40 micron sized particles or less to pass. This barrier can be breached as the result of several factors:

- Abnormal growth of otherwise normal lymphoid tissue cells (hyperplasia).[46] Cause: Vaccine over-reaction (autoimmune) to triggers like vaccine products. Measles vaccine virus is found in gut tissue in a high percentage of these children (also in spinal and brain fluids) (V.Singh, Uni.Utah, 2003). This is not so in seemingly healthy children, who have been vaccinated.
- Invasion by pathogens that produce enzymes to 'eat through' the protective mucus membrane barrier.[47] Cause: Antibiotics. Antibiotic resistant *stretpococcus* bacteria, *candida* yeast-forms and other pathogens multiply. These produce endotoxins (literally defecating in the bloodstream).
- Stress, allergens, heavy metals.
- Toxins from live pathogens (typically *Candida albicans,* but also bacteria) can also breach the brain barrier.[48]

Refined sugars can, in susceptible children, cause hyperactivity by stimulating a hyper-adrenal response.[49] This is not necessarily due to a 'leaky gut'.

Common pathway to ADHD

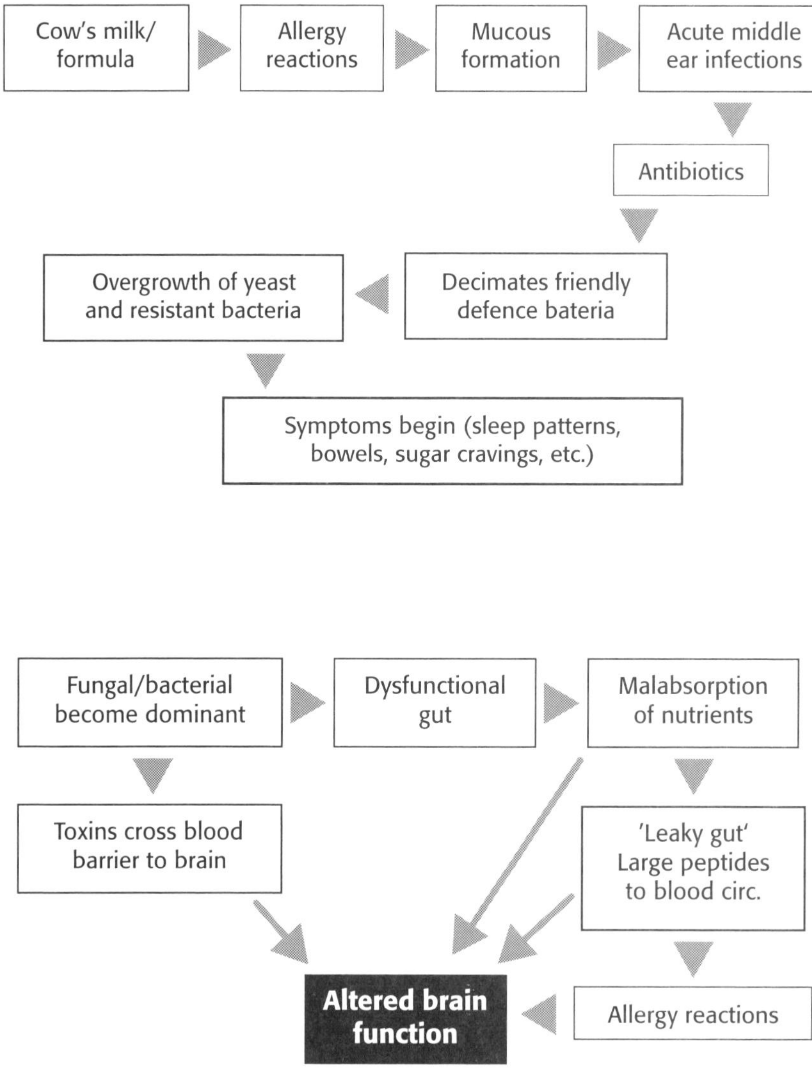

Behavioural problems such as hyperactivity, defiance, moodswings, aggression
Emotions unstable
Short term memory problems
Learning problems
Social instability

Parent ratings of behavioural effects of biomedical interventions

Since 1967, the Autism Research Institute has been collecting parent ratings of the usefulness of the many interventions tried on their autistic children.

The following data have been collected from the more than 22,300 parents who have completed the Autism Research Institute 's questionnaires designed to collect such information.

For the purposes of the present table, the parents responses on a six-point scale have been combined into three categories: 'made worse' (ratings 1 and 2), 'no effect' (ratings 3 and 4), and 'made better' (ratings 5 and 6).

The 'Better:Worse' column gives the number of children who 'got better' for each one who 'got worse'.

Parent Ratings – Drugs

DRUGS	Got Worse[A]	No Effect	Got Better	Better:Worse	No. of Cases[B]
Phenobarbiturates					
Prolixin	33%	36%	31%	0.9:1	87
Prozac	32%	32%	36%	1.1:1	1031
Risperidal	17%	29%	53%	3.1:1	471
Ritalin	45%	26%	29%	0.7:1	3650

Parent Ratings – Biomedical/non-drugs/supplements

	Got Worse[A]	No Effect	Got Better	Better:Worse	No. of Cases[B]
Vitamin A	2%	58%	40%	20:1	398
Calclum E	2%	62%	36%	14:1	1084
Cod Liver Oil	3%	SO%	46%	15:1	511
Colostrum	6%	57%	37%	6.0:1	213
Detox (Chelation)	3%	27%	71%	27:1	153
Digestive Enzymes	4%	43%	53%	14:1	413
DMG	7%	51%	42%	5.7:1	4725
Fatty Acids	4%	45%	51%	14:1	379
5 HTP	10%	58%	32%	3.2:1	81
Folic Acid	4%	55%	41%	11:1	1188
Food Allergy Trtmnt	4%	37%	59%	13:1	362
Magnesium	6%	65%	29%	4.5:1	295
Melatonin	9%	33%	58%	6.2:1	375
Pepcid	9%	60%	31%	3.3:1	75
SAMe	22%	54%	24%	1.1:1	37
St. Johns Wort	16%	62%	21%	1.3:1	61
TMG	15%	42%	43%	2.9:1	238

Transfer Factor	16%	54%	30%	1.9:1	50
Vitamin B3	5%	54%	41%	8.7:1	526
Vit. B6 alone	8%	63%	30%	3.9:1	599
Vit. B6/Mag.	4%	49%	46%	10:1	5284
Vitamin C	2%	58%	39%	16:1	1408
Zinc	3%	53%	44%	16:1	931
SPECIAL DIETS					
Candida Diet	3%	45%	52%	17:1	641
Feingold Diet	2%	47%	50%	21:1	666
GF-CF Diet	4%	33%	63%	16:1	933
Removed Chocolate	2%	49%	49%	30:1	1571
Removed Eggs	2%	60%	37%	16:1	949
Removed Milk Products/Dairy	2%	50%	48%	29:1	5159
Removed Sugar	2%	51%	47%	23:1	3486
Removed Wheat	2%	52%	46%	26:1	2842
Rotation Diet	3%	50%	47%	19:1	708

A 'Worse' refers only to worse behavior. Drugs, but not nutrients, typically also cause physical problems if used long-term.

B No. of cases is cumulative over several decades, so does not reflect current usage levels (e.g., Haldol is now seldom used).

E Calcium effects are not due to dairy-free diet; statistics are similar for milk drinkers and non-milk drinkers.

Birthing problems

In a small percentage of these children, their ASD syndrome can be traced back to birthing problems or later falls or blows involving the head. Clinics that specialise in ASD often use the services of practitioners who specialise in what is called 'cranial osteopathy' or 'cranial manipulation'. When born and while developing, the eight bones that make up the skull are surrounded by fibrous membranes that allow the skull to compress during birthing. As the infant matures, this is gradually replaced by bone.

In a Clinic in Australia, where I now work two days a week, we have the services of an osteopath who is trained in this method. He spent time in a Childrens Hospital in London where cranial manipulation proved very useful in a variety of childhood traumas and problems. These include autism and other ASD problems.

Cranial manipulation first began to be used in the 1930's, when it was (as most new and useful treatments) – very controversial. It was argued that the skull is 'fixed' – so how can it be manipulated? But the technique uses pressures and corkscrew movements that often achieve profound changes, especially in children who have had head trauma, and whose skulls are more 'pliable'. It is now a widespread speciality and the last five years have seen more research papers published on cranial work in osteopathic, chiropractic and dental journals than in the total of the last 65 years. An interesting example:

In 2001, a study using new electronic measuring devices graphically showed profound improvement in a subtle skull pulse named the cranial rhythmic pulse.

This pulsing is caused by the blood pressure and blood flow velocity. The subsequent 'wave form' of this measurement was seen to slow and regulate itself to a calming rhythm.[50]

Major food based autism/hyperactivity components – what they do

"The often quoted position that the relationship between diet and ASD has not been proven was based on research in the 1970's. It is now time to consider the useful studies of the 1980's and 90's that clearly show a relationship."

Joan Breakey M.AppSc
Journal of Paediatrics and Child Health, Vol 33, 1997

Some illuminating earlier history

The above landmark statement showed strong interest in the connection between diet and vaccinations in the generation of ADHD (and all ASD disorders). The next questions to be answered were:

- Why don't all of our children have such a connection? Are genes to blame?
- Why has this connection become so obvious in the decades following the 1980's?
- What other environmental factors cause our children's woes?
- Do these causes affect all the developmental disorders – because a high percentage of these children share similar symptoms?

The answer to the first question became apparent when it was shown that some children, like their parents, are more sensitive to environmental factors than others. This reflects a certain genetic component, but what caused this in the first place? It is seen that dietary and other health habits, plus results of generational exposure to environmental factors (as heavy metals, chemicals, vaccination) eventually cause functional problems that are followed, it is believed, by an individual genetic change. Several new childhood diseases have appeared in the last 30 years, that is, in the time-span when chemical and vaccination assaults have been the highest in the history of mankind. Typical of these non-inherited 'genetic' diseases is Smith-Magenis Syndrome (SMS) – first diagnosed in the 1980's, SMS has many of the symptoms that are common to nearly all the 'new'ASD diseases. This points to a common causation.

Another observation was that boys were four times more likely to be damaged by mercury and to develop autism, than girls. Fascinating new research has shown a slight increase in testosterone can increase Hg toxicity by 100%, whereas oestrogen decreases its effects.[83] However, girls do not escape so easily – a new rare disease, Rett's Syndrome (RS), which affects young girls almost exclusively, has become part of the 1990's pandemic of ASD. As in autism, the girl with RS usually shows an early period of apparently normal or near normal development until 6–18 months of life. A period of temporary stagnation or regression follows during which the child loses communication skills and purposeful use of the hands. Soon, stereotyped hand movements, gait disturbances, and slowing of the rate of head growth become apparent.

Other problems may include seizures and disorganized breathing patterns which occur when awake.

RS received worldwide recognition in 1983 when multiple cases were appearing around the world. **This is the precise period when the other ASD problems began to show an unmistakable climb following introduction of multiple vaccines.**

As in autism, the child regresses after normal development. As in autism, the serious symptoms are multiple and neurological. Although affirmed to be genetic, the following case clearly shows that environmental factors (in this case a vaccine) can mutate genes – which thus become only a secondary factor:

> "We report on a girl who, at age 2 months, developed an acute encephalopathy with destructive brain damage 12 hours after acellular pertussis vaccination (whooping cough vaccine). Months later, the girl manifested a Rett syndrome phenotype. DNA screening of the MECP2 gene was unrevealing in the child and her parents. This previously unreported association emphasizes the notion that Rett syndrome phenotypes can result from different (either genetic or environmental) causes."[51]

This case shows that vaccines can cause autoimmune diseases as found in the Autism Spectrum Disorders – in this case, Rett's Syndrome.

The next question to be answered was, "why have these problems become obvious during and especially following the 1980's?"

As mentioned above this was the time period when multivalent vaccines (three or more vaccines in one shot) began. This was also the time when ASD problems began to rise, dramatically.

What other environmental factors could be involved?

Firstly, the general level of the population's immune efficiency is declining. This was emphasised by the US Government experimental smallpox vaccine trial on 200 'strong and healthy' young adult students in late 2002. The results 'dumbfounded' even the Centres for Disease Control (CDC), directors of the campaign.

"The reactions we are seeing are totally out of line with today's vaccine experience and absolutely in line with historical experience," said Anthony Fauci, director of the National Institute of Allergy and Infectious Diseases. "In the 30 years since we have had routine (smallpox) vaccination, the public's tolerance level has gone way down."

Do immunised mothers 'pass on' immunity – as they once did?

Why has our 'tolerance level gone way down'? One serious consideration is the lack of immune system "priming" passed-on from our mothers because they themselves were in the generation when heavy vaccination was given in their childhood. Measles vaccination (single shots) began in 1970 (Australia). Those children are the mothers and fathers of the generation that began showing the worst immune performance period in our history for chronic immune diseases. Immunisation does not give life-time immunity, only natural "wild" infection does that. This may affect the parent's ability to pass-on to the newborn, natural immunity. That is a most serious consideration, one that will compound over time.

Asthma has doubled since 1982; some studies show 35% of children with this breathing problem. Over the same time period childhood brain tumours have increased by 50%. Middle-ear infections (acute otitis media),[52] once uncommon in young children, currently affect 80% of children. It now accounts for 75% of second visits to the paediatrician. Autism has risen from obscurity (approx. 2 children per 10,000), to be one of the most alarming signs of this pandemic.[53] Now one in 128 children have autism in USA according to Dept. of Special Education, 1999. Eleven new cases daily in California alone (2002). In the UK one child in 167 is now reported autistic. In Australia, 17 new cases weekly. This equates to one child in every 270 Australian children from one in 10,000 15 years ago! This maybe a low estimate. In my own experience (limited as it is in terms of investigative resources) at least one Australian school with 600 students has a special class for its six autistic students, and in the rest of the school "the teachers can't keep up with the numerous and growing population of ASD and ADHD children" (described by the mother of an autistic child I treat). This would equate to one in one hundred children with autism – in that particular location.

As to Question 3, other well-known environmental factors include lead and arsenic (which can cause ADHD & other neurological/ psychological symptoms), the increasing mix of numerous chemicals used in food and industry, and the also increasing use of antibiotics to which children have become profoundly resistant in the past decade. In fact, the school just mentioned is in an area polluted by surface coal mining (much airborne dust) plus agricultural spraying. Nevertheless, the local boy I am treating from there experienced serious side-effects from his vaccination program, and his regressive autism began to show shortly after. In those respects he is typical of probably 60% of all regressive autism.

Do vaccines actualy weaken immune systems?

There is a school of thought that the so-called 'minor childhood illnesses' of former times including measles, mumps, rubella (German measles) and chicken pox that entered the body through the mucous membranes, served a necessary and positive purpose in challenging and strengthening the immune system of these membranes.

According to the respected paediatric doctor, Harold Buttram, a presenter to Congress on vaccination issues, the respective vaccines of these diseases are injected by needle directly into the system of the child, thereby bypassing the mucosal immune system. As a result, the theory goes, mucosal immunity remains relatively weak and stunted in many children, complications of which may be the rapid increase in asthma and eczema now being seen, both in terms of frequency and severity.

This concept tends to be confirmed by four controlled studies, widely separated geographically, in which vaccinated children were found to have significantly more atopic (allergy) disorders than controls.

In commenting on the increased incidence of asthma and other atopic disorders in the United Kingdom in the article "Measles and atopy in Guinea-Bissau" the authors made the following statement:

> "The rise of allergic disease among children in the UK over the past 30 years remains unexplained.

"One hypothesis is that infections in early childhood prevent allergic sensitisation, and that successive generations of children have lost this protection as their exposure to infectious disease in early life has declined. Consequently the prevalence of atopy and concomitant allergic disease has risen."

It is true that in former times there were occasional serious complications from these childhood diseases, but this is an area in which nutritional approaches and homeopathy traditionally have been at their best. If these approaches were made widely available, it is probable that most of these complications could be eliminated. No one wants to see serious complications in our children, but the vaccine route may in time prove to be the worst possible choice that could have been made, as concerns the minor childhood diseases.

Threat of brain damage

Perhaps the greatest concern with vaccines today rests with their possible causal relation to the growing epidemic of childhood autism, developmental delay and attention deficit hyperactivity disorder (ADHD). Regarding the latter, a recent news item stated that ADHD has increased from 900,000 in 1991 to nearly 5 million today (in the USA alone).

At present, primary suspicion for this epidemic of neurobehavioral disorders rests with the MMR (measles-mumps-rubella) vaccine. Although scientific evidence has not yet reached the standards of scientific proof, one pioneer researcher in this area, Dr. Vijendra Singh with the Department of Pharmacology, University of Michigan, has published the report of a study in which he found that a large majority of autistic children tested had antibodies to brain tissue in the form of antibodies to myelin[55] basic protein, a protein strongly correlated to measles antibodies (almost all of the children had been immunized with the MMR vaccine, and none had had these diseases to naturally acquire these antibodies).

This study tends to confirm the results of a similar study published in The Lancet in 1998 by Dr. Andrew Wakefield and co-workers of the Royal Free Hospital in London, indicating a possible link between MMR vaccination, Crohn's disease of the bowel and autism.

Damage may yet escalate

"As another concept, it is highly pertinent that many of today's children are second-generation vaccinees; that is, they are born to mothers previously vaccinated with the measles, mumps, and/or rubella vaccines. It is possible that the reaction rates in the second-generation vaccines may be happening on a much larger scale due to previous sensitization of mothers from their vaccines, this sensitization being transmitted in turn to the foetes during pregnancy.

If this process is taking place, something we cannot know until appropriate research is done, there predictably will be additional increases in autism beyond that already taking place, and should the process be continued into a third generation. Time may prove that vaccine programs went awry when they deviated from the most basic of all medical ethics, the right of parents to accept or reject vaccines for their children". Harold Buttram is an author and physician at the Woodlands Healing Research Center in Quakertown, Penn. (Santa Fe, New Mexican, December 20, 2002).

Question 4 asked, "Do these causes affect all the developmental disorders – because a high percentage of these children share similar symptoms?"

Today, we know there are indeed connections in common and new pathology is showing that the ASD's are not primarily an illness of the mind but unwellness in the gastro-intestinal tract (which in this book, for convenience, we will call 'gut') that causes brain dysfunction.[56,57] Because autism is the most serious of the child development problems, it is (rightly) the most researched. Its statistics are known. But autism casts a long-shadow, and these sometimes 'lesser' problems (ADHD, Aspergers, and ADD etc) are seen to follow the trends found in autism itself. The symptoms are less, but many of them are common to all ASD children.

The gastro-intestinal link

The common thread among the majority of children suffering in this wide-spread epidemic is bowel flora disruption and inflammation in the gut (dysbiosis); in many children this includes overgrowth (dysplasia) of the immune system glands surrounding the gut.

World-wide research of these problems over the last eight years can be summed up by this extract from the June 2002 Harvard University/ Massachusetts Children's Hospital Study of 600 ASD children, headed by paediatric gastro-enterologist Dr Tim Buie.

> "More than half of these children had treatable gastrointestinal problems ranging from moderate to severe … these children are ill, in distress and pain, not just mentally, neurologically dysfunctional," said Dr Buie. "They were treated successfully by replacing

suspected gastric enzyme and probiotic deficiencies. The results have been significant improvements in the patients' conditions."

Dr Buie noted that both the physical and behavioural symptoms improved in these autistic children. This extensive study added strong evidence to the many years of work done around the world in treating ASD's via gut improvement. This work has been ignored and denied by the conventional drug oriented pharma-medico industry.

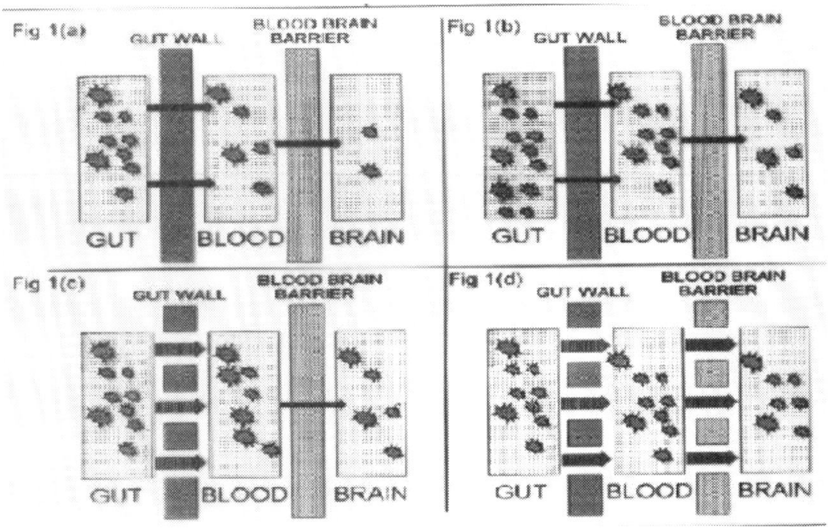

From Sunderland University (UK), Autism Research Institute School of Sciences

This endeavours to illustrate how oversize food particles (peptides) can pass through a 'leaky gut' wall, enter the bloodstream and then pass through the blood/brain barrier to cause behavioural and other brain dysfunction. Called 'intestinal permeability' in pathology, this 'leakiness' can be identified by new laboratory techniques at a low cost.

The GUT disruption genesis for ASD's was the same conclusion that I had come to in 1999 when commencing the treatment of suspected ASD problems. In a study of my first 57 children, I found 82% of them reported stomach pains and gastro-intestinal problems. I began to treat these symptoms, with which I was very familiar – having specialised in the naturopathic treatment of gastro-intestinal problems for 30 years. To my surprise, and the parents delight, we found so-called neurological/psychological problems began to dissipate. Hyperactivity, in more than 95% of cases, disappeared or became easily manageable inside of a few days. However, the older the child the more often we found that the hyperactivity had become a habit rather than a physical/mental imbalance (usually after 12 years of age). Although hyperactivity was now no longer itself an uncontrollable force, sometimes the behavioural habit itself had to be retrained. But usually the young person desired to break this habit (they had lost their friends, self-esteem and lots of school learning through it).

Common physical symptoms in ADHD
Study of 57 children
(Sichel 2000)

Condition	Number	Percentage
Bowel dysfunction	48	84
Stomach pains	45	79
Poor sleep	42	74
Sugar cravings	40	70
Itching	31	54
Very smelly stool	25	44
Thrush (females)	22	38
Skin rashes	21	37
Vaccination effects	15	26
Food sensitivities	14	25
Bed wetting	13	23

The discovery that a high percentage of these children and young people (and men in their twenties) could lose their apparent ASD disorder symptoms by treating the gut function, showed what Dr Buie's Harvard University team had found in 2002, autism/ADHD "behaviours and actions were potential symptoms of intestinal complaints". Those findings represent incontrovertible evidence from yet another impeccable source confirming that Autism Spectrum Disorders are not primarily genetic, nor a brain problem – but in the large majority are environmentally caused via damage to the gut.

The significance of these findings is high, on two counts:

- At least 1000 children are being diagnosed with autism annually in Australia and autism is only a part of the wider spectrum of ADD and ADHD, Aspergers and other pervasive development disorders (PDD's). Combined, we are looking at a major childhood pandemic. (Imagine, if 1000 children were to be diagnosed with meningococcal annually, 10% may die but 25% would have neurological damage similar to autism. What an outcry there would be. We have at least 17 children weekly diagnosed with autism in Australia – yet how many of us have heard about that?)

- Most of these problems are being dealt with using pharmaceutical drugs with known side effects. These drugs are aimed at the brain not the gut.

In regard to numbers, we are showing the same history among our children as the rest of the developed world. The comparative silence about this pandemic will be discussed in more depth later in the book (see Chapter 14).[58]

But first, we must discuss the current advancing (non-Government/ pharma industry) treatment consensus of this epidemic.

CHAPTER FOUR

Natural treatments

Instant information for parents with little time

This Chapter contains a reasonably comprehensive outline of the many natural and biologically scientific steps that can either completely or partially restore most ASD problems. We either use these methods, or – in cases where we see the need for expertise outside our own field, refer to practitioners so trained.

Repair of ASD is necessarily a comparatively new and certainly fast growing science – brought on by the several environmental challenges described in earlier Chapters and faced by today's child. Therefore, new science discoveries are announced almost daily from prestigious institutions around the world. I have tried to keep up with them to this date!

Note for do-it-yourself parents

It is important to understand that although these methods may appear simple, there is a genuine need for you to see a practitioner who understands functional medicine and all its ramifications. This is not said to 'drum-up business' (as some may say) – unfortunately there is altogether too much of that anyway. We wish it were so simple. But repairing ASD/ADHD damage requires skill and experience. For instance, in use of vitamin B6 and magnesium (mentioned in this Chapter) – sometimes 'huge' amounts are needed before a result is obtained. These amounts most parents would never dream of using. Also, as by way of example, even moderately high use of B6 only (without extra magnesium) could bring on convulsions. There is also the matter of selection of the correct therapy for the individual. Even twins can differ here.

So, I recommend you take time to read this Chapter through, as it cannot be properly summarised. Then you will understand what your selected practitioner is talking about and be able to co-operate intelligently.

Full explanation of natural treatment of Autism Spectrum Disorders

This includes information for 'distant' clients not able to personally attend our Clinic. Many clients have been restored this way. See also Appendix Eight, 'Questionnaires'.

As you have read in 'Causes of ASD's', a damaged gut is heavily implicated in nearly all of the children with ASD's. Because of this well-known problem, a growing number of pathology laboratories have developed specialised tests that carefully analyse the several important ways in which a malfunctioning gut can go wrong. These pathologies are examined in more detail in a following Chapter. They play an important role in helping us to more carefully plan a recovery program specifically tailored to your child's treatment. Many of these tests, plus heavy metals (mercury, etc) and nutritional deficiencies, attract a Medicare rebate.

New pathology and new treatment bring ASD/ADHD reversal

However, before most of these new tests first became available many thousands of children were being restored or totally cured by wise doctors and naturopaths around the world using mostly dietary and biological methods. Some of these doctors and naturopaths are household names among the ASD communities.

This new approach has arrived just in time. In 2000 the US Congress was given evidence that methylphenidate (Ritalin-type drugs) can change brain chemistry permanently, and can predispose a child to future cocaine abuse. The evidence also included profound changes in the delicate interrelational and 'humanity' faculties. Some children were found to lose a part of their natural ability to socialise, to explore and be curious, and to play. In a 1999 retrospective study (*Canadian J. Psychiatry*) it was found that nine percent of ADHD/ADD children on methylphenidate developed psychiatric problems. None of those not taking the drug developed any psychosis.

Because of their willingness to break away from the drug approach and explore therapies that will address the causes and not the symptoms of our damaged children, many of the physicians who developed the natural approaches are regarded as heroes by parents of recovered children.

From among the most famous of these practitioners we have chosen some whose work you can follow-up on websites or in books they have published. For those who wish to do this, please see the Appendix. Probably the best known is Dr Bernard Rimland, founder of the Autism Research Institute in America. He is the father of a talented young man with autism. In the 1960's Dr Rimland wrote a landmark book which successfully challenged the then common view of the medical profession that autism was the fault of what they called 'Refrigerator mothers'- mothers who failed to show love to their child. Rimland showed that autism was a biological function problem not a psychological problem. His thesis changed the attitude of the medical world towards parents and their autistic children.

Today, with increasing knowledge, we know that it is indeed not the mothers who cause the problem of late-onset autism, but in most cases inappropriate medical interventions.

Working with other like-minded physicians he began using several specific dietary changes, lifestyle factors and restorative biological therapies. Today, we owe a great debt to the pioneering work of these men and women.

In 1985 I started using some of these therapies in our Fountaindale Clinic. This new direction began after meeting with Dr William Crook, one of the American paediatricians who worked along the same lines as Bernard Rimland. 'Billy' Crook, as he was affectionately known, became another household name among ASD and candidiasis affected families. He wrote many useful books and also the landmark book *The Yeast Connection* (and he wrote something for the back cover of this book). His quite simple methods have helped in clearing most of the problems suffered by my child-patients and, in the case of children with hyperactivity or ADD, offered a safe and effective alternative to drugs. Later, after more precise pathology became available, I began to work with autism – using the same methods with added biological medicines that can in various ways restore both gut and brain function (neurotransmitter messaging). As the American paediatric gastro-enterologist Dr Tim Buie has noted, "both the gut and the brain share the same need for the same nutrients" and have other features in common. One of my recent serious autism cases is described below (and appears on the video available in conjunction with this book). His case is typical.

If you take the time to carefully read this case and see what happened, then you will be a long way towards understanding how this treatment works and how we restore both gut and brain function.

A story that illustrates a typical treatment

The Story of Brock

Presented at the Clinic on January 8 2003, brought to me by his mother Colleen, and father Stephen. He was 2 yrs and 10 months.

Had been diagnosed by his paediatrician as Autism Spectrum Disorder. His parents wished to avoid medical drugs.

Brock had developed his collection of autism-like symptoms immediately following a later than usual triple-antigen vaccination, at 3 months of age. On the same day he began to scream uncontrollably, this lasted for seven days. He went "blue & limp" at two different periods over two weeks. He was hospitalised twice. These episodes are known as Apparent Life Threatening Episodes or A.L.T.E. *Paediatricians admit* (at least among themselves[60]) *that both ALTE and SIDS deaths are commonly associated with vaccination adverse events.* Brock's episodes peaked on day 5 and day 12 post-vaccination. According to several studies[61] those days are among a group of critical days in the dangerous three weeks post-vaccine period for major flare-ups. In fact, his worst ALTE (when his condition was serious) was day 12, known to be a time when both immune defence and body exhaustion sets in. He was hospitalised both times.

Before this, Colleen said, he had been a dream baby – sleeping well, happy, affectionate, normal bowels and digestion. No skin problems, no symptoms at all (except for a runny nose at 2 months, which caused his mother to delay the vaccination, agreed by the paediatrician). But Colleen had intuitively felt he should not be vaccinated at all.

Immediately after this adverse event, Brock began a list of increasing regressive symptoms, typical of the most common form of vaccine related regressive autism-type disorder. No longer a dream child, these problems now included a lack of his usual affection, cessation of eye-to-eye contact, 'stiffening' and not agree to being lifted from his cot or pram, bowels became alternating loose an hard, reaction to certain colours, 'rocking' in his cot and hitting his head against a chair, and aggression – long and often with tantrums

Possibly the most lethal of all was a TIA (a transient stroke) that left Brock with some paralysis of his left side plus imbalance. Fortunately, his mother worked with physiotherapists who showed her how to restore him. Today there are no visible effects of the TIA.

Brock became 'very, very destructive' – he would destroy toys and books. He sniffed everything and had other obsessions – especially with garbage bins. He would follow the truck down the street (no stopping him), he would replace lids that were open, try and right bins that were thrown over, right round the streets. He would listen for the garbage truck. It became a grave concern to his parents. Other obsessions included absolute demand that their water fountain be kept going at all times.

My findings

Because of his condition and multiple symptoms, I ordered a Complete Digestive Stool Analaysis (CDSA) that also included a search for pathogenic bacteria, yeast forms and parasites. This was commenced on his second visit, on January 24.

On his first visit I also tested his zinc level, which was at the lowest point measurable.

As with nearly all these children, he had sugar cravings and multiple allergies that included cow's milk, penicillin and yeast.

Treatment

As usual, I changed his meal times so that his major meal was breakfast and included protein. He had another protein based meal at lunch, and his evening meal was vegetables only, or soup or gluten-free porridge (polenta) or gluten-free wholemeal cereal or crispbreads and avocado or similar. These all digest easily and quite rapidly. With this program his sleep began to improve (although for a few days he had nightmares – his body was changing, for the better). An initial reaction to treatment is common in children, for him it was so for every change. Fortunately, Colleen recognised these changes (which in Brock's case often included 40 °C fevers) for what they were – good events. On my advice, she did not try and suppress the fevers. She told me that after every period of these fevers yet another permanent improvement manifested. His case is most illustrative of what is called Hering's Law – a law of the order or progress that takes place in natural healing, where fevers are a friend, not a foe (see Chapter on Fever in this book).

His initial remedies included:

- *Digezyme* enzymes – to help his gut digest food better and more completely.
- *Intestamine* – a powder that helps the gut to repair (for older children we use *RejuvenX*). These are produced by Bioceuticals, a company specialising in ASD.
- *B-Vital* powder – supplies high dose B vitamins, minerals and amino acids.

- *LifeStart* bacteria – the *bifido bacterium infantis* probiotics that repair and protect.
- *Zinc Drink* – to replace his zinc deficiency. Zinc is a major trace element in neuromessaging. I test all children for zinc because nearly all ASD children are deficient.

Later, these were added:

- *Nylstat*, an anti-fungal – after the CDSA revealed a high level of *candida glabrata* (a fungal yeast) in his gut. (For older children, who can swallow capsules, I give a product that contains a New Zealand herb called *Horopito*. This has equivalent 'kill' ratio to any of the powerful anti-fungal drugs. Or citrus seed extract, which must be taken with care, with advice from a practitioner.)
- *Hepato-D* – for a suspected bile problem. This is a homeopathic remedy.
- *CP* & *PPMP* from Blackmores for nerves & calcium.
- *Essential fatty acids* – effective for higher intelligence quota and reduction of hyperactivity, depression, aggression and impulsiveness.

Brock was also taken off all sugars (including fruit, except one apple) – replacing the sugar with *Stevia*, herbal drops that are 30 times sweeter than sugar (but with virtually no calories – which feed the gut pathogens). He was given vegetable juices made from carrot, green apple and spinach. This was also the 'vehicle' for his medicines.

Outcomes

In the first sixteen days, Brock began to improve. His bowels normalised (after a short period of 'mega-diarrhoea' – Hering's Law at work), his tantrums did not last as long, and he began to concentrate better. He was calmer. His appetite really began to improve.

Today, 3 months after treatment began, Brock is a new boy. He is no longer destructive; he shows affection and looks at you directly with his eyes. He plays with people, like any little boy – but still has traces of compulsive activity, occasionally 'the needle gets stuck in a groove'. His aggression is far less and far shorter – getting better as the treatment works. His Autistic Association worker, who visits regularly for sessions, says he has changed so much since the treatment began; it is now possible to interrelate normally with Brock. His speech is much improved, but there is a way to go here.

However, he still sniffs things, his social skills need further improvement, and his garbage bin anxiety is now localized to the family bin! He no longer needs to have the fountain on. He has just turned three, and my prediction is that by four years of age any residual condition will be indiscernible.

A closer look at why the treatment worked

How is it possible for eye-contact, social skills, affection and so many other 'brain' things to change so dramatically by taking common bread, milk and sugar out of the diet, killing off some common gut yeast and adding a few simple nutrients?

Many have asked that question! I remember the father of an autistic boy whom we treated successfully who told me that when he heard about this 'no bread' method he said, "What a lot of nonsense!" Below is a picture that tells a thousand words.

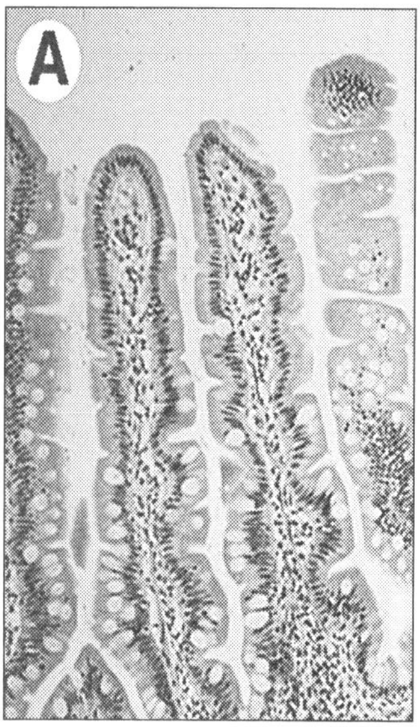

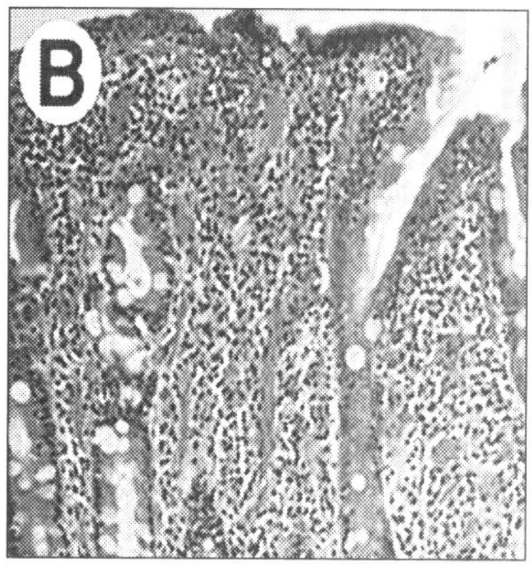

A shows normal small intestine villi, the 'fingers' through which digested food nutrients are absorbed into the bloodstream.

B shows villi damaged by untreated gluten intolerance in celiac disease. Gluten is bread protein.

Celiac & ADD both same behaviours and GF diet response

Several researchers have observed ASD behaviours in Celiac Disease (a gluten intolerance disease):

"Emotional symptoms are common in children with celiac disease, although they are not often the initial mode of presentation of this condition. Children with celiac disease have been described as 'extremely irritable, fretful, capricious or peevish. Nothing seems to please them and although they are quite unlike themself.' They often exhibit features of extreme emotional dependence on their mothers, frequently clinging to them and showing marked irritability and fretfulness when separated. In addition, they are often emotionally withdrawn from their environment, and this withdrawal may even resemble autism. The association between celiac disease and autism is still a matter of considerable debate in some circles."

From a speech by Ivor D. Hill, MD. Professor of Pediatrics, Duke University entitled Clinical Presentation of Celiac Disease in Children, *given on July 14, 1995*

"The effects of the gluten-free diet are most often spectacular, particularly in toddlers. Behavioural disorders are the first to subside ..."

From Coeliac Disease, by Dr. Michael Marsh Blackwell Scientific Publications, November 1992, Chapter 2 (by Jacques Schmitz), p.30

"Psychological changes have also been widely investigated, but are difficult to quantify. Many patients appear to be depressed, while others are irritable, morose or difficult to relate to ... Nevertheless, in some case reports, treatment with a gluten-free diet has resulted in spectacular improvements in mental function."

Ibid, Chapter 3 on CD, written by Peter Howdle and Monty S. Losowsky. p.55

We will tell you more on this later, but first we will look at the frequently found yeast problem.

Maybe we should let the pathologists speak. Pathology is the science that can find the 'why' behind unusual clinical success. Without such 'proof' western medicine will not consider taking on a new therapy (and if it is not a drug or patentable, it will usually still not take it on).

The pioneer pathologist in the field of autism spectrum disorders has been Dr William Shaw, director of the Great Smokies Laboratories. While working at Children's Mercy Hospital, the paediatric hospital for the University of Missouri, he became interested in the role of abnormal levels of urine organic chemicals called metabolites while evaluating two brothers who had autism as well as occasional muscle weakness. Previously, he had worked for the Government Centres for Disease Control, and used the then new investigative tool named 'Gas chromatography- mass spectrometry' (GCMS), which enables a pathologist to see peaks and valleys in quantities and types of body chemicals, with speed and accuracy never known before.

In a famous interview, Dr Shaw had this to say.

> "When I first started in this field, the analysis of a single chemical compound would have taken most of the day. Since then, we can identify a thousand different compounds in a single afternoon."

This technology had never been applied to study abnormal organic body chemicals in autism before.

> "Since some inborn errors of metabolism are associated with muscle weakness, I was really looking for metabolites (products of body chemical activity) characteristic of these conditions which were all negative. Instead, I noticed that several unusual compounds were consistently elevated. None were adequately described in the medical literature.
>
> Colleagues in the field of metabolic diseases said they were probably from gut flora (micro-organisms). Since several of these compounds were analogs (altered forms) of normal energy production (Krebs cycle) compounds, I thought these compounds may be significant, perhaps as anti-metabolites.
>
> At the same time, I was testing the culture media of a large number of different yeast and bacteria strains from the human gastrointestinal tract in order to find out which compounds in the human might be derived from the yeast and bacteria.
>
> During the same time period, I began a collaborative study of evaluating urine samples of patients with schizophrenia obtained by Dr. Gattaz at the Central Mental Health Institute of Germany in Mannheim.
>
> These samples were very valuable since they were obtained from patients who were drug-free. Thus, any biochemical abnormalities would be due to their condition and not a drug effect."

A child with an acute psychotic reaction had been tested when relatively well and then was tested again during the psychotic reaction had a much higher level of a compound derived from tyrosine (an amino acid) during the psychosis than when he was well. A colleague in the field suggested that this compound was derived from micro-organisms in the intestine.

> "The compound that was elevated in this child during the psychotic episode was also found in a large percentage of the

adults with schizophrenia. Since tyrosine is the raw material used by the body for the production of neurotransmitters, I suspected that this product might be very important."

This finding showed a strong connection between psychotic disease and autism and abnormal conditions in the gut.

Later, Dr Shaw found another significant metabolite that showed another connection between the gut and autism.

The compound that led to the discovery was tartaric acid. It is a known toxin that inhibits cell energy production, and reduces brain function. Humans do not produce this chemical. The only source of tartaric acid is yeast, and is known as tartar in the wine-making industry – a sludge produced by yeast activity fermenting the grape sugar.

The brothers with autism and severe muscle weakness had extremely high values of tartaric acid in their urine. Another child with autism had a urine value of tartaric acid 600 times than that of normal children.

Dr Shaw then examined the medical charts of several other children with autism, they had similar abnormalities and immediately he saw a possible causal connection. He was aware of Dr William Crook's clinical discovery that treating for yeasts cured many behavioural disorders.

"The next step seemed obvious. If these compounds were from yeast and were causing some of the symptoms of autism, antifungal drugs which kill yeast should reduce some of the symptoms of autism.

At that time a two year old boy was currently being evaluated for autism at the hospital where I worked and I had just done the organic acid test. The child had been developing normally up to about 18 months of age and had a vocabulary of 100 words. He was treated several times for ear infections with antibiotics and developed thrush (a Candida or yeast infection of the mouth and tongue).

His behaviour deteriorated quickly after that. He lost all speech, became extremely hyperactive, woke up all night long, lost eye contact with his parents and was diagnosed with autism. His organic acids that I thought were due to the yeast, including tartaric acid, were very elevated. The neurologist at the hospital would not prescribe the antifungal drug Nystatin for the child so the parents and I convinced an outside paediatrician to prescribe it. The child's eye contact returned by the following day and the elevated organic acids decreased markedly, although it took 60 days to return to the normal values.

I have found that these metabolites are not specific for autism but may also be associated with other neurological conditions such as ADHD, seizures, learning disabilities, or speech disorders. In one set of identical twins, one of the twins was autistic while the other was not autistic but had speech difficulty.

The factors that influence which condition is present probably include which metabolites are elevated, how high their concentrations are, how long the exposure to these products lasts, the number of exposures, and differences in the ability to detoxify these products."

With Brock, as with so many of my children, the initial rapid improvement came as a result of taking away the sugar that fed the yeasts (*Candida albicans*). The gradual improvement came from the slow repair of the gut with the specialist nutrients and bacteria. I then prescribed the simple to take liquid 'Nylstat', to speed up the anti-candida process. From there on, he began to rapidly improve.

Later in this Chapter I will share with you the new pathologies and the newly discovered herbal treatments we now use to combat candidiasis. 'Nylstat' is a useful drug, with no side effects, except with prolonged use it can cause the *candida* to migrate through the bowel membranes into deeper layers, where the yeast buds can 'hide' to begin again once the anti-fungal levels reduce.

A closer look at additional neurotransmitter biologicals

These help the brain cells to communicate with one another

To repair the brain damage caused by these toxins we use several potent neurotransmitter supplements. These include special vitamins and minerals in high amounts.

I will begin by sharing with you some of the exciting and proven results using vitamin B6 and magnesium; zinc and dimethylglycine (DMG) (a derivative of B15)- and the amino acid glutamine, all important neurotransmitter enhancers found in a healthy person, but often lacking in ASD's. Vitamin B6, for instance, is essential in neurotransmitter metabolism. It is very often deficient in ASD studies. Glutamine, removes the waste product ammonia from the body. Zinc is an essential brain signal agent. Both zinc and glutamine are also typically deficient in ASD.

However, too much B6 can cause seizures, but only if magnesium is deficient. When we give children very high doses of B6 we also include large amounts of well absorbed magnesium. The results can be spectacular in autism (see ARI panel, page 29).

Too much zinc accumulates in damaged brain tissue (for instance, from a stroke) and can accentuate the problem in adults – but not so in children, who seem to need lots of zinc.

Orthodox psychiatrists and paediatricians laugh at the concept of such simple nutrients bringing any change at all to such problems as ASD's. But, using comparatively large amounts of these simple nutrients early researchers found significant results among the diagnosed autistic children with whom they worked. There was better eye contact, fewer mood swings, improved speech and less self-stimulatory behaviour ("Stimming", as it is called, includes spinning in one spot, rocking, banging the head against walls etc). The children became more normal, showing interest in the world around them. Any change for the better, however slight, is a landmark for the parent of such a child. And these are much more than slight changes.

As I was writing this, a mother phoned me from interstate. Her five year-old boy had slowly been experiencing some 'windows' of improvement in treating his autism. Now her voice sounded very happy and relieved. The last two days had seen him speaking descriptively (with adjectives), carrying on a conversation with a neighbour's child and asking dad to make a hop-scotch pad on the patio. He even began to trial the hop-scotch (with low/medium results!). These were unique events for him. They were all suddenly the best 'window' of improvement yet. They followed the introduction of DMG, B6 and magnesium only one week previously. Prior to treatment, the boy had been regressing and was becoming a great worry both at home and at school, where teachers were complaining of his behaviour. These improvements, in only 11 weeks, meant so much to both his parents and himself, that happiness was beginning to reign. The boy himself had so much wanted to improve (but couldn't because of the chemical chaos in his brain) that he took all medicines as well as he could; only complaining over one of them.

Phased introduction of treatments to assess viability

There are today numerous biological methods and remedies we use to treat ASD. They can often be used together, several all at once, in what is called the "shotgun" approach. It is very tempting to do this, as we know there will be a beneficial response in most cases. But this does not allow us to see which remedy or nutritional change has made some progress in the child. Nor does it allow us to find the specific remedy if the child reacts adversely. I hasten to add, these events are very rare and very mild using these methods. Just some diarrhoea or vomiting, with no lasting result. They usually indicate a highly toxic child who needs slower progress and cannot begin to be compared to the frequent and often frightening list of side-effects from drugs.

Too much was just right!

Dr Bernard Rimland is fond of recounting the story of the American mother who visited the group home of her autistic adult son. She was horrified to find his behaviour gains on the B6 program had crumpled. They had run out of his 1,000 mg per day supply. She immediately ordered three times the usual amount of the B6/magnesium powder, so he wouldn't run out again. On her next visit she was amazed at his unprecedented improvement. He actually showed her affection for the first time ever! She later found out they had mistakenly given him 3,000 mg daily, three times the normal dose!

Postscript: the physicians in charge later stopped the B6 formula, despite his improvement – it was "dangerous" they said. And gave him a truly dangerous drug instead.

In regards to the amount of B6 and magnesium, this is often a question of "how much is enough?" and this can vary greatly from person to person, depending on their current ability to take-up the nutrients from the gut. This itself is a reflection of the degree of gut disorder (dysbiosis) they have developed. A practitioner can help by using his experience and also some tests can be run.

My first use of these nutrients, plus special dietary changes – which we will look at in depth later, proved interesting. He was a seven year old autistic boy, diagnosed at Sydney's Westmead Childrens Hospital. The dietary changes brought instant (five days) improvement in behaviour and happiness. His parents noted him laughing for the first time, and becoming more 'part of' the family – showing the beginnings of normal responses.

Later, we added the B6 and magnesium supplements plus B complex (giving B6 on its own may cause numbness and other neuronal symptoms because any gross B vitamin imbalance has its own problems). This is what the family then noted:

Day-by-day further neurologically based improvements began to surface. He began to play with his sister, he "settled down", and was able to perform 'motor' events he could never have done before.

Gluten casein sugar-free – the classic 'GF-CF-SF' diet

Once again, orthodox medicine heaps ridicule on such a simple measure to treat such (apparently) complex problems as ASD's. And once again, the evidence is in – and has been for a long time.

Gluten and casein are both proteins. The former is the principle protein of most grains (except corn, buckwheat, millet, rice, quinoa and amaranth) and the latter that of milk and the basis of cheeses.

In the long-term study of 724 ASD children by Dr Bernard Rimland, using the GF-CF Diet, he found 64% got better, 33% had no effect and only 4% appeared to worsen. This result confirmed the suspicions of several research groups around the world (in the 1980s) that undigested food particles (peptides) may enter the bloodstream via a 'leaky' gut and cause the behavioural changes seen in autism disorders. These researchers had found these peptides in the cerebro-spinal fluid of some people with autism. Later, the University of Sunderland (UK) Autism Research Unit found these substances in the urine of 70-80% of people with autism. Opiates act like morphine in the brain, and the researchers believed that some of these food particles were able to cross the blood-brain barrier and disrupt normal brain function. It is well known that casein (from human or cows milk) will break down in the stomach to produce a peptide known as casomorphine which, as the name implies, will have opioid activities. Similar effects are noted with gluten from wheat (and the gluten cereals barley, rye, spelt, triticale, kamut, farina and oats, although some can take oats without problems) in which case the compounds formed are gluteomorphins.

The fact that 64% of over 700 hundred got better on a CF-GF diet is a startling proof that the gut/brain natural barriers are breached in many ASD children. These results tended to confirm the Sunderland University study in which they found such peptides in the urine of 70-80% autistic people (but not normal people). This percentage was almost the same as the Rimland results with symptom improvement (64%).

Today, the CF-GF (often, if gut dysbiosis and hyperactivity is present, I add SF – sugar-free) is standard practice among those of us who treat ASD's with natural methods.

In my practice I have seen these results over and over. But let me tell you a story of how 'modern' medicine regards this approach.

The father of one of my clients attended a conference organised by the Autistic Society in Australia. During the conference he stood up and told how his son had improved so much on the GF-CF diet. The lecturer replied to him, "We are not able to recommend such a diet to our clients, sir." Later, during lunch, that same lecturer came up to him and said, "If I had a child with autism, I would certainly put him on a GF-CF diet."

In contrast, another client was advised by a medical specialist to 'increase his Coca Cola levels'. So, Coke's OK, and Ritalin, amphetamines and many other mind altering (and sometimes damaging) drugs manufactured by the pharmaceutical companies are OK – but not a gluten-free or milk-free diet! Oh, no. That is 'too simple – how can it work?' Oh, and also there's no money in it.

Milk protein *casein* hits the current affairs TV programs

While writing this section, two popular 'current affairs' broadcasters ran a controversial story on milk protein (casein). They reported on work done by the New Zealand Dairy Research Institute that found two forms of beta-casein, Type A1 (found mostly in Friesian cows) and Type A2 (Gurnsey and Jersey cows). Type A1 caseins were found to be involved in heart disease, Diabetes Type I (insulin dependant) and autism spectrum disorders. The 'nasty' beta-casein was designated as BCM-7 (beta-casomorphine-7). This binds to brain cells via morphine receptor sites on the cells.

I decided to search for more information and came across a previously restricted New Zealand Dairy Board memorandum that showed a lengthy history of international research going back to at least 1993. This had shown a distinct relationship between Type A1 milk protein and the morphine-like symptoms in ASD children, and also in schizophrenia. An American study found that no less than two thirds of ASD children had elevated casomorphines (BCM-7's) in their urine, which was not found in the general population of children. That means that probably two thirds of autism spectrum disordered children have at least some morphine-like behavioural effects. (The BCM's were also not found in the general population of a NZDRI study).

This vital information was published in a medical journal, but never made it to the ones who needed it the most – our children. What a wonderful chance it would have been to have greatly improved the life of tens of thousands of ASD children. If the public report had been released earlier (when the facts were conclusive), then it would no doubt have caused a disruption in the dairy industry. However, this could have been controlled if carried out in a sensible manner. It would probably have saved thousands from going into Diabetes I and would certainly have helped tens of thousands of ASD children live a far better life.

It was during digestion that Type A1 was found to release this bioactive peptide called beta-casomorphine (BCM-7). The NZ Dairy Board Research Unit also collaborated with other international scientists on studies that showed two-thirds of ASD children were affected by these

BCM's. This exactly parallels the early work (1996) at the UK Sunderland University Autism Research Unit that found casomorphines in the urine of autistic and ADHD children. As described elsewhere in this book, casomorphines can enter the brain of children with a 'leaky gut' and pass through the blood-brain- barrier to cause 'morphine-like' affects on the brain. The report also noted that this effect was widely known then among scientists. Note: it is still denied (2003) by most paediatric medical authorities! Why? Because drug companies make money out of the effects of Type A1 milk on children, (and also on gluten containing foods – like bread, which release their own morphine-like substance). They prescribe reactive drugs to try and counteract these effects.

But also there was evidence of its effect on Diabetes Type I (insulin dependant), and also hyperactivity. You can now buy Type A2 milk.

A farmer breeding prize stock knows exactly what the foods and specialist nutrients will do in those precious bodies. Today's top athletes rely on extensive nutritional programs to achieve optimal condition, including tests for 38 trace elements; recognition that physical performance is affected by the quality of the food consumed. Meanwhile, people often choose to eat foods that are deficient in vital nutrients and allow their children to eat food-less junk, and consume food and drink that is positively harmful. As parents, we must also consider mineral and nutrient discrepancies.

Not only champion stock and athletes need a base of proper nutrition to be fit and healthy; we all do! In fact, of all mammals human beings need a greater range of some nutrients than any other, including:

- Essential fatty acids that predicate our IQ, found in large amounts in human milk but only as traces in cows milk, and
- High zinc levels, a trace element related to motor (movement) performance, reading ability, neuropsychological function, immune function and hundreds of enzymatic total body reactions. (Almost 98 percent of my child ADD/ADHD patients are zinc deficient!)
- More than 60 other trace elements

Good trace element nutrition can help prevent killer viruses

The importance of trace elements was highlighted by a recent US laboratory study of a common, relatively benign influenza virus (the so-called Bangkok virus) which mutated into a serious pathogen in laboratory mice that were raised on a diet deficient in the trace element selenium – a powerful antioxidant. The discovery, according to the researchers, demonstrates a unique mechanism by which viruses can mutate and points to the importance of antioxidant protection against viral diseases. The selenium level in the study's deficient diet was one-sixtieth that of the adequate diet. From my experience with selenium levels in numerous hair analyses, it is often borderline in my patients.

A previous study by University of Carolina virologists Melinda A. Beck and BHNRC nutritionist Orville Levander reported that a strain of coxsackie virus mutated from mild to severe in selenium-deficient mice. Could the SARS virus have been stopped by adequate selenium? Maybe.

Benefits of human milk

Mother's milk is the absolutely best product for babies! In fact, medical authorities warn that cows' milk should not be given to infants under a year old. Goats' milk, unlike cows' milk, presents few of the problems and in many respects – although higher in protein and lacking 'BB' – is close to the qualities of human milk. It still contains casein, and therefore sometimes may not be so good in the CF diet. However, this is usually after other immune lowering events have caused a problem. If milk supply is short, and supplementation looms, try fresh goat's milk first.

Although Type A1 casein in cows appears to have the worst effect of any milk on ASD, it must be remembered that even human milk contains casomorphines, which can affect the moods of both mother and infant. But these are usually positive effects. It appears that not until the child sustains auto-immune damage from vaccines do Type A1 milk casomorphines (and the equivalent peptides from gluten) begin their devastating effects. This has been demonstrated by a lack of morphine-like opioids in the normal child/infant population.

A mother's milk has the right mix for a human baby: the right amount of protein, calcium and iron, and especially in early feeding, fine globules of easily digested fat. The iron, particularly, is highly bioavailable. The bioavailability of all the nutrients in mother's milk is believed to be the reason why comparatively small amounts of some nutrients are found compared to other species.

Also, antibodies and bacteriostatic (bacteria-stopping) proteins in breast milk can reduce the risk of disease, including the common middle ear infection in a child, for years. Even diseases like lymphomas, Diabetes Type I, and Crohns disease. But this is sometimes offset, unfortunately, by the power of vaccines and antibiotics to damage children. Many of them come to me with a good breast-fed history yet later (after the first triple-antigen shots or antibiotics) they begin, usually, with a series of otitis-media (mid-ear infections) or other problems.

Only human milk also contains factors vital to our children:

- Essential fatty acids (EFA's) that have been shown to have a significant impact on intelligence levels of infants, and are now widely believed to be an essential part of the reason why human IQ is so high compared to animals (cows have virtually nil EFA's). Such deficiencies maybe made up later in formula-fed babies, when solid feeding commences, but development delays can be expected.
- Even in studies as late as eight years after birth, earlier infant breast feeding (which always contains EFA's) found significantly higher intelligence scores, compared to children on formula in early infancy. But, as with folate, the baby will suck mother dry of EFA's and it is essential for her to eat adequate unrefined carbohydrates, which are linked to fatty acid production. It has been also suggested that mothers should supplement with EFA foods, especially the long-chain variety (e.g. as found in eggs and fish).
- Sources of EFA's: vegetable oils (sunflower, olive, soybean corn); nuts and seeds; and long chain fatty-acids in sardines; herrings; mackerel etc.
- 'BB' factor molecules enhance the growth of friendly Bifidobacterium bacteria (*B. infantis, B. longum* and *B. bifidum*). Depleted *B. infantis* can now be regained by use of powders made from cultured live *B. infantis* species.

However, it is vital to remember that the mother's life-style and eating habits are reflected in the milk. For instance, some specific vitamin and mineral supplementation can advantageously increase these vital nutrients in a mother's milk. These include B6, adequate vitamin C, folate, manganese, iodine and selenium. But not without a consultation from an expert in this area. For instance, iodine should be added very carefully. Excess vitamin C does not reflect in the milk, which maintains a normal level – but the mother needs to make sure she is taking enough herself. And there is no problem with taking too much – only temporary diarrhoea will occur (cured by reducing the vitamin C). Adequate folate (folic acid) is still needed after pregnancy, as the infant literally sucks it out of mother – even to the point of mothers own deficiency (so, that tells us something – infants need particularly sufficient folate!). The same applies to essential fatty acids.

Folate is also the best sun protector. Take or (later in his development) give your child adequate folic acid, B12, zinc and Vitamins C and E – and you'll be protected better than with sunscreens, says the renowned American doctor Jonathon Wright MD. He calls folic acid deficiency "a major contributor to skin cancer risk," and he adds, "Folic acid is destroyed rapidly by heat, cold, and exposure to light, including sunlight. So it's sunlight's destructive effect on folic acid in the skin, not the actual sun exposure itself that accounts for a significant part of the skin cancer problem. Folic acid (along with vitamin B12 and zinc) is the absolute key to DNA reproduction and repair."

The best dietary sources of folic acid include spinach and other dark green vegetables, brewers yeast, lima beans, cantaloupe, watermelon, wheat germ. Also, liver from organic farm bred animals.

Dr Jonathon Wright has serious doubts about sunscreens. He cites a 2000 study carried out by the Norwegian Radiation Protection Authority, which showed that low doses of octyl methoxycinnamate (OMC – the anti-UV ray ingredient in almost all sunscreen products) killed mouse skin cells. Research suggests that OMC may be toxic to human skin tissue as well.

Having said good things about mothers milk, it must be remembered that heavy metals like mercury and lead are now also almost universally found in mothers milk, but in greatly varying quantities (e.g. from 1.50 µm/dcl lead in country areas to sometimes 45 µm/dcl – in some women in Mexico City). The same applies to smoking (nicotine etc), alcohol, recreational drugs and marijuana. Mercury (Hg) from amalgam fillings, the most serious source of Hg, can also contaminate the foetus.

Eating too many big fish may be a mercury hazard

Eating Hg containing fish is another frequent culprit, e.g. shark, king mackerel, pink salmon (red is OK) and swordfish are among the worst.

However, two average size fish meals a week of the smaller varieties was considered 'safe', according to an FDA 'Advice to Pregnant Women' (2001). Or two tins of tuna a week are OK.

Another American institute screened 720 patients from March 2000 to March 2001, then tested the mercury levels of patients who reported eating ***more*** than two servings of fish a week.

The tests showed that of 116 patients who had their blood tested, 89 percent showed mercury levels greater than the 5 parts per million recognized as safe by the National Academy of Sciences.

Of that group, 63 people had blood mercury levels more than twice the recommended level and 19 showed blood mercury levels four times the level considered safe. Four people had mercury levels 10 times as high as the government recommends.

The study monitored 67 patients as they reduced their fish intake and subsequently their bodies' mercury levels. Within 41 weeks, all but two had reduced their blood mercury levels to below government-recommended thresholds, according to Hightower.

This was an American study, and it should be remembered that Americans are fond of the larger, longer living fish – which contain most Hg.

Was FDA fish study a red-herring?

But the above fish studies may prove to be a red-herring for most of us. The study below, published in *The Lancet* (a prestigious British medical journal) and confirmed by the American John Hopkins University Hospital, tell us that pregnant mothers do not have to be concerned about a reasonable fish diet. Indeed, the above FDA study maybe using fish as a scapegoat! The literature is full of evidence showing both the American and British Establishments are trying hard to find other reasons than vaccines for the undoubted presence of excess mercury in autism spectrum disorder children. So far, they are not succeeding. Fish has recently been in their spotlight. So have power stations. Even mercury amalgams – but never vaccines!

The *Lancet* results confirm earlier findings that prenatal exposure to mercury in the Seychelles – where fish consumption is the main component of the local diet – is not associated with impaired neurodevelopment in young children.

A research team from the University of Rochester, USA, with colleagues from the Seychelles investigated 779 mother-infant pairs enrolled in the Seychelles Childhood Development Study. Mothers reported high fish consumption – 12 meals a week compared with one meal a week on average in the USA. The fish in Seychelles contained similar concentrations of methyl mercury as commercial ocean fish elsewhere. Prenatal Hg exposure was determined from maternal hair growing during pregnancy.

The investigators assessed neurocognitive, language, memory, motor, perceptual-motor, and behavioural functions in children at nine years of age.

Dr Constantine Lyketsos from Johns Hopkins Hospital, Baltimore, USA, concluded, "On balance, the existing evidence suggests that methyl mercury exposure from fish consumption during pregnancy, of the level seen in most parts of the world, does not have measurable cognitive or behavioural effects in later childhood...For now, there is no reason for pregnant women to reduce fish consumption below current levels, which are probably safe."

The questionnaires

Having read all about various factors that can damage your child you may be wondering exactly how your child has been affected by these events. Finding that out is the first step in the Treatment Plan, which starts with one or two questionnaires (see Appendix 8). Later, we may suggest one or more of the special pathologies now available (see Pathology, Chapter 7). These will pick up precise evidence of both the presence and severity of any pathogens and/or damage to the gut or liver functions.

The questionnaires have been carefully constructed from the findings of a multitude of previous families who have been there before you. Questionnaire 1 deals with the total history and current symptoms of your child, while the other questionnaire, is a quick version of one designed by the Autism Research Institute and gives an indication of the category of ASD in which your child most closely fits. This helps to plan the road back to normalcy, and gives an indication of what to expect.

Each question is very significant to us, even though some may not appear to be so to you. So, please answer them carefully and fully. They provide a picture of the current state of your child and also the history that led to this condition.

Once completed, we are able to quickly hone in on the significant signs and factors and question you further and more precisely.

These signs and factors include early signs of vaccine reaction, significant use of antibiotics at any age, but especially in early infections, caesarean birth, birthing problems, premature births, milk intolerance, sugar cravings, food allergies, bowel and gut problems plus the learning and behavioural problems. There are many other factors, as you will see in the questionnaires, but these are the major signposts. Some can only be answered by pathology – that means, testing of stool or urine by a laboratory that specialises in ASD research.

One of the first major efforts in the Treatment Plan is a quick reduction of troubling symptoms, which may include stomach pains, alternating hard/loose bowel motions, poor sleep, hyperactivity, and what one American parent calls 'Ooops, wrong planet' children. That is, the spaced-out, not-with-it, doesn't-hear-me child with significant damage.

Making friends with your child

Without the co-operation of your child, the job of recovery is a more difficult road to travel. Fortunately, most children are very keen to co-operate. They just don't want to be where they are at present. They have very often lost their friends, cannot co-ordinate, are low in the class, can't read very well (if at all), feel miserable and unwell and suffer from various discomforts. Because of these frustrations they go into major tantrums or become withdrawn. Of course, there are a myriad variations of these difficulties and behaviors.

For me, making friends with these children (or older ones) is the best part of my work! I know how they feel, and tell them that I do. I speak with them directly, as 'man-to-man', and they appreciate that – and listen. Of course, there are the extreme ASD's, ADHD's and ODD's, and very young children with whom it is not possible.

One important visual tool I use is the 'Evil Empire' chart(see next page). Although it deals with just one of the problems that seriously affect many of the children, and cause many of their woes, it can be adapted so they understand the importance of 'chasing the Enemy out of their tummies' by not feeding them sugars. The Evil Empire chart shows *Candida albicans* yeast forms enlarged 7,000 times (7K), on which we can draw an unpleasant face! It also shows a cross-section electron microscope photo (40K) of the body wall of one yeast bud. This names the various types of glyco-proteins (sugars) from which their bodies are made. We call them 'bodies made of sugar'.

The question is asked, "What do you think they live on, Johnny?"

Johnny thinks ... and thinks.

Sometimes the matching concept is too much for him. Other times, he may answer 'sugar', with triumph in his voice. If it's been too much to work out, I say, "Why, they live on sugar, because their bodies are made of sugar" – and the light turns on.

Then we have him in our conspirational plan to 'destroy the enemy' – NO sugars anymore! Use of this method is also possible for distant clients, but best done by someone from outside the direct family who is respected by the child – like a grandpa or an aunt; or it can be done by a person not known to the child.

You would be surprised how powerful this simple tool is to get a total 'no sugar' program going. Johnny has made this decision – he sticks with it.

But we help the program to succeed by giving the herbal sweetener Stevia to take the place of sugar. It is 30 times sweeter than sugar, and has no or hardly any calories. That means it will not feed yeasts, or streptococcus or any other pathogen that needs sugars.

The success of this strategy is important (because sugars are a real poison in these children – as in all children – as you will read elsewhere in this book). Here is a story to show how well it works.

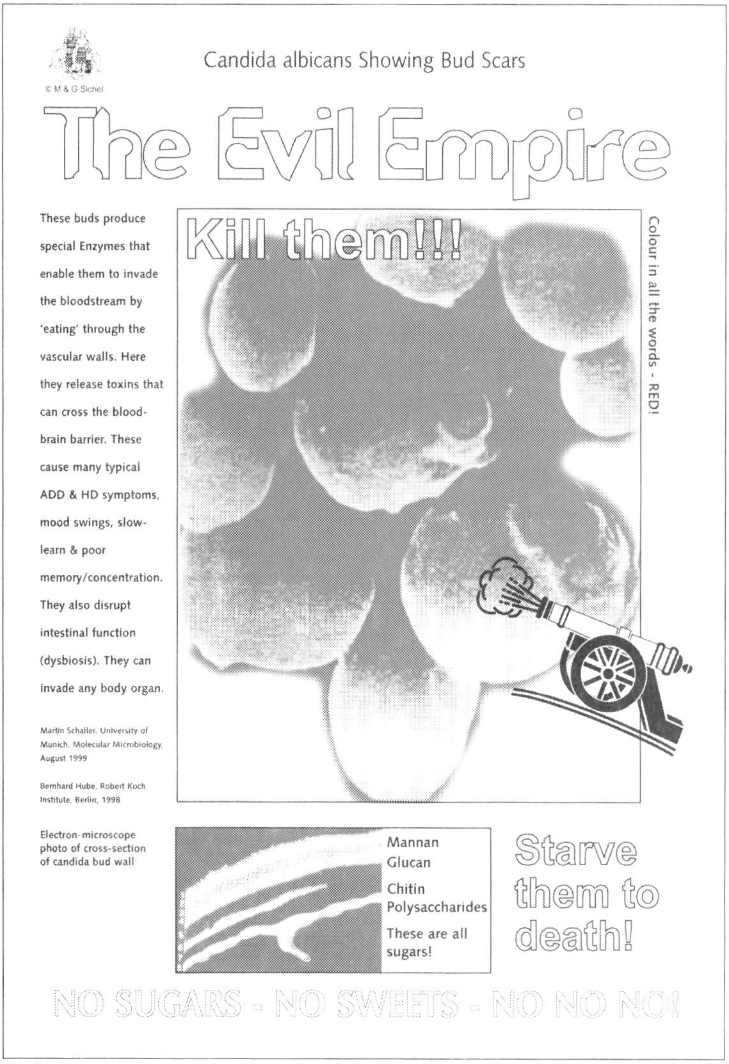

Candida albicans Showing Bud Scars
© M & G Sichel
The Evil Empire
These buds produce special Enzymes that enable them to invade the bloodstream by 'eating' through the vascular walls. Here they release toxins that can cross the blood-brain barrier. These cause many typical ADD & HD symptoms, mood swings, slow-learn & poor memory/concentration. They also disrupt intestinal function (dysbiosis). They can invade any body organ.
Martin Schaller, University of Munich, Molecular Microbiology, August 1999
Bernhard Hube, Robert Koch Institute, Berlin, 1998
Kill them!!!
Colour in all the words - RED!
Electron-microscope photo of cross-section of candida bud wall
Mannan
Glucan
Chitin
Polysaccharides
These are all sugars!
Starve them to death!
NO SUGARS - NO SWEETS - NO NO NO!

"Have some jelly beans," said the doctor to the child. "No thanks", she replied.

The mother of one of my young female patients went to the doctor after a week or so on the treatment regime for a check up. The mother had been very happy with the progress and so had the little girl. The girl had left my office clutching the standard 'Kill the Enemy' chart in her small hands. She had the usual determined look on her face *not* to feed sugar to the enemy *anymore*!

Her mother described to me how the doctor had told her that "candida certainly could not be causing ADHD symptoms" – and offered the little girl the usual handful of jelly beans.

My little patient, however, obviously thought otherwise and said, "No thank you, they will feed the enemy!"

She said this because she *knew* why she was feeling much better.

However, I decided it was time for more definite scientific proof that candida could, indeed, cause both ADHD, ADD and many other of the problems I had seen clear-up so many hundreds of times over 15 years by treating obvious candidiasis infection. If there was evidence around, I was determined to find it (see Chapter 8 for more information).

Our experience shows that we must treat *Candida albicans* and associated pathogens (such as *Candida glabrata*) in a large percentage of these children. This infection can begin in one of three major ways, over-use of antibiotics; cross infection during birthing; vaccine auto-immune response (upset of humoral/cellular response).

Another example of candidiasis damage

On Monday July 8, 2000 the popular *New Idea* magazine published an article on the work of myself and other naturopathic clinics and doctors using similar methods in the treatment of children with ADHD.

Some 300 families contacted either our clinic, the Australian Natural Therapists Association or other clinics. In fact, our clinic phone became too busy and we had to transfer calls to our home. The parents said they did not want to use drugs or wanted their children off the drugs and that they had tried 'everything'. The very first family to see me travelled from Sydney on that Wednesday.

I later wrote the following to the *New Idea* journalist who had interviewed me in the first place:

> … my very first patient from your article, an unhappy, but otherwise lovely little 5-year old has done so well. Her mother rang me with delight only *four days* after treatment began and said her daughter had slept through the previous night for 'the first time in two years' and that 'yesterday she was playing happily *with other children*' (she had become totally unsociable) and 'now she is playing happily by herself on the carpet in a corner of the room'.
>
> Another young current patient: an 10-year old ADD boy who I began to treat a month ago. His teachers were sceptical about our

methods. The mother told me that her boy is reading and learning so well now that the teacher has asked what exactly is happening."

I remember how happy I felt for that first little girl, she had been so miserable only a few days before. What that mother had said was very significant. She had unknowingly listed the positive reversal, **in four days**, of the commonly reported and damaging effects of metabolic toxicity caused by *C. albicans* yeast-forms infection, which will be conclusively proved in this section, supported by evidence from research, clinical trials and experience from prestigious international Institutions. Here had been a typical ADHD child, mood-swinging, unsociable, uncomprehending, restless, disinterested, 'disconnected', miserable (plus pale, sleep-problems, stomach-ached, 'itchy and bitchy'). In four days transformed into a normal, happy and beautiful little child! What had made this change?

From then until now we see this same outcome with remarkable consistency.

On December 2, 2000, *New Idea* published a letter with photos from another family, two more of my recovered children. These were two brothers, aged eight and eleven. Their mother was a teacher.

Despite finding that treating candidiasis brings positive results, a very good pathologist whom I know, told me recently that his laboratory has not found a significant number of candidiasis results in patients. A doctor who works closely with this pathologist told me, however, that antibiotic-resistant *Streptococcus* was found in significant numbers. She said that these *strep* infections also feed on sugars.

However, I found in studies during 1985 (on 67 patients) at our then live-in naturopathic hospital, that using drug antifungals (like Nylstat) over periods of time can cause the yeast to migrate through the bowel walls into the deeper tissue.

Here it 'hides' until the Nylstat danger is over. Then it breaks out again. This maybe the answer why yeast infections inevitably return after drug treatment and why pathologists cannot always find abnormal populations in the stool.

But either way, treating these infections with a sugar-free program will bring results.

We also now use the oil pressed from grapefruit seed (grapefruit seed extract) to treat not only *Candida,* but also *Streptoccocus* and most other gut pathogens, including larger forms like amoebas and parasites. It works very well and mostly does not harm our friendly bacteria. It is a powerful natural medicine and should only be prescribed by a qualified person.

Summary of treatments

First consult

Questions answered
Pathology suggested
Inhouse tests (zinc; blood alcholol etc)
Other diagnostics, iris diagnosis
Nutritional changes to lessen immune load
Education for child & parent on causes and repair
Initial prescriptions – gut repair, digestion improvements,
Initial brain improvers – neuro-transmitter nutrients
Osteopathic diagnosis (cranial, neck, spine)

Second Consult

Pathology discussed
Additional treatments, to suit pathology results
Progress discussed
Questions answered – usually menus, food etc

Ongoing Consults

Progress reports
Further fine tuning of treatment
Later (about 3 months) pathology repeat for assessment

Biological medications (summary)

Natren's LifeStart powder (*Bifidobacterium infantis*) as directed, for children and infants under 7 years of age.

Note: If you ever have to use antibiotics, give LifeStart after the course to replenish the friendly bacteria in your child's intestinal tract. Two weeks' use, two teaspoons or more daily.

For children and adults over 7 years, use Natren's TrenevTrio, or dairy-free DFA. Always make sure that you buy your friendly bacteria from the fridge at your health food shop.

Daily use of Eleotin for blood sugar control.

As prescribed

DMG (di-methyl glycine) – neurotransmitter
L. glutamine – repairs both gut and brain
Phosphortidyl-serine – brain function
Transfer Factor – the ultimate immune system enhancer: powder can be taken from capsule and used in vegie juice, if necessary. The more acute and long-lasting the problem, the higher the intake. Even

hourly. TF is harmless and has no side effects. TF turns the immune system on to its best fighting mode. Take daily until improvement. Infants: one capsule, separate from capsule and add to breast milk or formula being used. babies over 3 months, two separated capsules. Children: up to eight caps daily (for acute problems). For Caesarian babies or babies not breastfed: always use TF – the contents from one capsule daily for five days from birthing, spread over feeds. Do not give capsule container (the gel). Apply to infant with finger, in mouth or in breast milk. Always use Transfer Factor in place of antibiotics

All the supplements below can go into vegetable juice. warm water, soy milk, rice milk or a little goat's milk (unless your child is very lactose and/or casein intolerant).

B-Vital powder – a B and amino acid complex
Zinc Drink – easy to take in drinks
Note: Most children with these problems are zinc, magnesium and essential fatty acid deficient. The importance of zinc cannot be overemphasised for ADD, autistic or slow developing children. Eighty percent of our little clients show zinc deficiency. The forebrain has the majority of what are termed zinc containing neurons. Zinc is directly related to motor performance, reading ability and neuropsychological function (*Journal of Nutrition*, 130;2000).
Essential Fatty acids – essential brain function improver
Vitamin C – essential immune system nutrient
Hawaiian Pacific Spirulina – for natural complete nutrition
RejuvenX – an excellent gut repairer
Intestamine – similar to RejuvenX
Xenoclear – for de-tox
Digezyme – treats stomach pains caused by 'gas', reduces flatulence, assists food absorption
SAM-e – methylation improvements
Selenium – antioxidant and therapy for allergies
B6 – brain function
Magnesium – all these children are magnesium deficient

Other specials may include, sleep remedies, homeopathics, stomach improvers, multi-phasic magnet therapy and many other 'tools of the trade'.

Also, referral to learning and behavourial therapists – usually after the physical symptoms subside (which cause most of the child's discomfort and malfunction).

Foods to eat in candida-induced problems

You child maybe prescribed a gluten-free and dairy-free diet for a few months. ***Therefore, some of the guidelines below will not apply.***

Follow the candida diet, and do not force things – just take it easy, and use your wisdom to introduce these changes to your child. It has taken time for your child to become unwell or hyperactive, but following this program, most children respond so fast you will find it hard to believe!

Meal Reversal

Breakfast

Principle = protein.

This is essential if you wish to make it easy for your child to give up sugars of all kinds – cordials, sweets, fruit, honey, etc – which are 'feeding the Enemy'. This means you will have to make breakfast your main meal for the day. (Don't panic! Please try this for one week – you will be delighted with the results.) You will eat your protein for breakfast, plus vegetables or salad. Your child will sleep better, not be so hyperactive during the day, will not crave sugary things, will behave better, be more restful, happy. The bowel movements will improve (if there are current problems).

If possible, always follow breakfast with plain yoghurt. Use carob powder (tastes like chocolate) for taste, or ground sesame or sunflower seeds (no husks!). Sesame is fifty percent calcium, and both seeds are rich in essential fatty acids. Use Jalna bio-dynamic yoghurt.

Lunch

Principle = protein. Maintains blood sugar levels evenly.

Use one 100% wholegrain bread, read the labels, and remember, 'the whiter the bread the sooner you're dead!' is not just a funny rhyme – there is much truth in it. It is said that white bread is only healthy for the breadmakers! They profit in providing the least nourishment and lots of air. Try pushing one of those sliced whites together end-to-end.

You will be left with less than 2 centimetres of actual substance! If you read 'bakers flour' on the labels this equals white flour, even if the bread is 'multi-grain'. You can eat rye bread (100%), but yeast-free bread is best. Sour dough is okay. See your health food shop (HFS) for 'Essene bread'. These breads cost more, but they are worth more too.

Many good breads are now available at the supermarkets and health food stores. One of my favorites is 'Bill's Bread'. Made from stone-ground organic flours, this bread is raised with sourdough, so contains no baker's yeast. Children usually like its sweet and nutty taste. ('Bill's Bread' consumer services number is 02 4942 1042 – Newcastle, NSW.)

Another source, this time gluten-free, is Uncle Ricks GF Foods, see their website www.unclericksglutenfree.com or call 1800 100 970. They deliver all over Australia.

Use 100% full-grain crispbreads like Ryvita or Vitaweet (unless on a GF diet), rice cakes, etc.

Try your child on alternative spreads, like almond or cashew nut butters, or Swiss 'Tartex' (HFS). Use freshly made peanut butter (HFS) or Sanitarium natural peanut butter, plus salads with cheese (use good cheeses if possible, not Kraft etc, which are full of food chemicals). Try Dutch Edam or Gouda, or Tasmania Mersey Valley (very tasty cheeses), or Bega – sharp or mild.

Evening meal

Principle = easy to digest light meal.

Soups or porridge made with soya milk from millet meal and oats (or barley) in winter. On porridge use sesame seed and/or sunflower seed (no husks!) ground into powder in electric coffee grinder, blender or similar. Use freshly made on porridge or in plain yoghurt. Use crisp-breads, salads, avocado and yoghurt for summer.

To make a vegie juice cocktail use washed, fresh, raw, unpeeled carrots, celery, beetroot, greens of all kinds, plus green apple. Drink twice daily.

Do not give any cow's milk! Use fresh goat's milk, or soy/rice milks or the vegetable juices you make fresh. Cow's milk lies behind many illnesses in children. Your child will not become calcium deficient!

Stevia is a natural sweetener derived from a herb and is thirty times sweeter than sugar with only two calories per serve. Stevia does not feed candida or cause intestinal fermentation, and it has a positive effect on the stomach and digestion.

'Kids' Favourite' homemade lemonade recipe (sugar-free)

Use always in place of other soft drinks. Slice 1 lemon and the ½ lime. Soak in pure water (not tap water), for 24 hours. Juice the second lemon and add to sliced lemon/lime water. Sweeten by adding Stevia, one drop at a time, until required sweetness.

If your child wants his usual soft drink bottle, just save one and fill it with your homemade Kids' Favourite lemonade.

CHAPTER FIVE

Meet the kids

Children and their brave parents who came through with flying colours

Every ASD child is different! Because the individual immune system is part of the uniqueness of us all, every child responds more or less strongly and in his own peculiar way to every environmental challenge. The American autism parent association, Autism One, puts it this way:

> "Biomedical treatments have proven to be effective in correcting many of the biochemical imbalances found in children with ASD. Many children suffering from acquired autism, for instance, exhibit biochemical disorders ranging from intestinal dysbiosis, to disproportionate levels of vitamins and minerals, to elevated red blood cell counts. Each child, however, is unique. Each child's requirements are different.
>
> Algorithmic 'one-size-fits-all' approaches generally do not work. Rather recognizing the diversity, multiplicity, and sensitivity of each child is necessary. Imbalances, although patterns are evident, are not always treated in the same way."

The same facts apply to all the diseases in the ASD spectrum. There is no 'one-size-fits-all' among ADHD kids either. I wish there was, it would be far easier to apply treatment, and parents could virtually do it all themselves. But, experience is required and skill in choice of both the type of pathology and therapy required.

So, you will find a wide range of problems presenting in the children below. That is the way each has responded to an environmental assault – often, a medical intervention. Below is a list of common findings among Alphabet Kids:

- In nearly 35% of severe cases a reaction to vaccination is seen prior to onset
- The child has "regressed" – what had been learned is now being lost or spoilt
- There are gastro-intestinal symptoms (bowel problems, stomach pains)

- The stool, and often excessive flatulence, are unusually odorous
- Dark eye circles
- Line wrinkles just beneath the lower eyelid
- The child rubs his/her nose upwards, cheeks and ears get very red
- The last three signs indicate the allergies/food sensitivities common to ASD
- *Candida* induced skin problems, itching, migrating sub-dermal lumps
- Sleep patterns are poor, e.g. the child cannot get to sleep or wakes frequently
- There has been a significant history of antibiotics
- This history centres on middle-ear infections and respiratory problems
- He has a sugar addiction/craving
- He wets his bed (enuresis)
- She has been exposed to lead, mercury, chemicals or other toxics
- There has been an unusual pregnancy/birthing
- Plus the many familiar behavourial/learning problems, which are actually *symptoms* of some of the above physical malfunctions (as noted by Dr Tim Buie in the Harvard/Massachusetts General Hospital collaborative study, 2002).

You will see indisputable evidence in this book that at least 80% of these children have somatopsychological problems (body affecting the mind). This is not a strange concept – one only has to remember someone in the family whose poor liver function caused tiredness and depression, or whose sugar addiction always ends in hyperactivity. Now scientists have found how gut problems can cause long-term (chronic) mind/learning/behavourial problems. We prove the connection daily in our clinical situation.

It is also true that we find no cases of 'Ritalin Deficiency' among these children! Furthermore, of what use is it to give a chemical drug that alters the brain function, when the brain is being disrupted by events taking place in the gut?

Yet, 50,000,000 medical brain stimulants were prescribed to children in 2000 (*Sydney Morning Herald)*.

Occasionally, in cases of severe Opposition Defiant or severe ADHD children, we find that dexamphetamine should be continued until the natural treatment begins to normalise brain and behaviour function. And this can certainly help.

But the long term use of these medical drugs can sometimes cause addiction and worse. I recently read of a woman whose 30-year-old son had been treated with Ritalin for several years as a child. But in his late teens and continuing as a young adult he turned to street drugs. On being questioned he said that they made him feel more like when he was taking Ritalin. Later, after he finally managed to cease the drug habit, he suffered from depression, couldn't hold a job, and struggled to keep normal relationships with others.

Certainly, this is not an isolated case. The recent release of an eight year prospective study on hyperactive children using amphetamine-like drugs showed 80% of the children still with ADHD. Worse, 60% had deteriorated to the extent of now being diagnosed with the behavioural disorders Opposition Defiant Disorder (ODD) and Conduct Disorder (CD). Now, the possibility of long-term side-effects is being raised (does that sound familiar?). In the United States, between 1990-1997, 2,993 Adverse Reactions were reported, including 569 hospitalisations and 160 deaths (FDA Division of Pharmacology Report). Bearing in mind that only 1–10% of Adverse Drug Reactions are reported (according to the FDA), these are devastating statistics.

Positive stories of natural restoration

Here are the stories of nine different types of ASD children, plus a teenager and a young working man. Eight of these came to our clinic and, over only a few months, were either totally or significantly restored. Maybe you will find your child's problem among them?

The ninth is a boy from another country; he was treated in much the same way, and serves as an example of the world-wide success in treating ASD without drugs. By searching the net for 'autism spectrum disorders' you will find thousands of other examples.

In most of these cases, the Alphabet problem came on them well after birth. This damaged them severely, and their plight and behaviour affected their parents and grandparents – and their brothers and sisters. The wonderful news is that these children are closed to being totally restored or vastly improved.

1 My first Alphabet family (1993)

By mid-June 1993 Mrs S of Killarney Vale, NSW was beside herself. She had three boys with health problems. Of one she said, "David is a total problem – 90% of the time just bad". He refused about everything – from dressing in the morning, going to school, learning, eating, speaking and being nice in the day to undressing and going to bed at night.

Another of the three boys was anxious to learn but couldn't. Tom just was not able to concentrate, was always fidgeting – hyperactive and unhappy (ADHD).

His mother first brought Tom to our Fountaindale Clinic.

My notes, made at the time, read, "Tom is a friendly and willing boy. He desperately wants to succeed. This is not just a behavioural thing, there must be an input problem here, probably something he is putting into his body – or not putting into his body."

I began the work of discovering what the factors were. By changing his diet and adding certain nutrients Tom changed in just a few days as was evident by two school 'Awards for Concentration' in the first week.

Then Mrs S. brought the Bad Boy to me. After a week, she came back with David and said to me, "He has been WONDERFUL! I cannot believe it! Now he is 90% good and only 10% bad!"

This story is not exaggerated. How these amazing changes took place is of course the subject of this book.

2 The story of Joshua

Joshua's mother and the school teacher cried with happiness! "It was as though somebody had turned the light on," said the teacher.

Note: Joshua was one of our distant clients. He lives within flying distance, not driving distance! We never came face-to-face, and all consultations were by questionnaire, phone and email.

Joshua's mother phoned in the last week of March, 2003. She had read an article on our work with ASD in *Classroom*, a journal for teachers.

Her son was 5 years of age. Because of a pregnancy complication (polyhydramnios) he had been born prematurely, weighing only 1965 grams, with a forceps delivery.

Between three and four years of age his parents noticed he was not developing normally. He was also developing obsessions over certain routines and would grind his teeth. His walking, running and balancing were poor. Other symptoms included some 'stimming' when frustrated (head banging and spinning).

At school, his teacher had become very concerned for him. Joshua was worsening. He was 'lying around all the time'. In the classroom he would lie on the carpet, apparently very tired and obviously lethargic. He was sometimes exhibiting irregular behaviour, 'almost drunken-like'. His eye contact deteriorated, he did not interact with family or friends, did not join in with school activities, and was a most unhappy little boy. His speech was significantly behind, and learning was very slow. But he had unusual skills with numbers, puzzles and jig-saws.

Joshua's mother and father had become alarmed at his behaviour. In fact, when his mother phoned her voice was one of quiet desperation.

She was sent a copy of our ADHD Questionnaire (which you will find in this book) by email.

Investigations

Later, we organised a Complete Digestive Stool Analysis, an Intestinal Permeability Test and a hair analysis (Joshua lives in a town somewhat contaminated with industrial hazards, including arsenic).

Treatment

The first step I took was to send Joshua's mother digestive enzymes, essential fatty acids, and child intestinal bacteria, and Metagenics Zinc Tally to test his zinc levels. He was also placed on a gluten-free, casein-free diet. I also requested that his mother (who works in a pharmacy) buy Nylstat, an anti-fungal, to help reduce what I believed was a gut-born yeast infection.

These measures caused some improvement in a few days, but his mother was still very concerned, as the major symptoms had not improved.

As the various pathology results were not yet in, I worked through the Questionnaires, phoned her again for more clues and as a result sent her a magnesium replacement therapy, vitamin B6 high dose, a fortified B vitamin powder. A few days later I sent her dimethyl-glycine (DMG – an efficient neuro-transmitter enhancer).

On April 9, Joshua's mother phoned, very excited by major improvements – she told me that Joshua had begun talking with adjectives (descriptive language), had asked to play hop-scotch and was even having conversations with children at school.

When the pathology results were all in, we found Joshua had:

- A "leaky gut"
- Hypochlorhydria (low gastric enzyme/acid production) & resultant maldigestion
- Putrefactive phase digestion
- Above normal arsenic level, boron beyond highest limit
- Essential minerals imbalance and four trace elements undetectable
- Among them, significantly, Lithium was undetectable (sodium levels were normal)

On April 15, to adjust some of this functional and nutritional pathology, we added:

- Lithium (Li) orotate (which is non-toxic). Lithium supplementation can reduce excitable and restless symptoms when given to those who are deficient.
- Fullhealth Australian colloidal minerals – which supply 70 trace elements
- Bioceuticals 'RejuvenX' – a most effective gut repair nutrient powder
- Remedies, taken before meals, to increase gastric output
- A homeopathic for stomach function
- Organic Spirulina, total nutrient supplement (less Vit C) and gut flora enhancer
- Reducing his meat levels drastically, replaced with other protein, countered putrefaction quickly

On April 30, we had a wonderful call! Joshua's mother phoned in crying – with happiness! Joshua had been back at school. After the two weeks holiday his teacher had seen wonderful changes in him. So much so, that when his mother arrived, she found the teacher in tears – of relief and joy).

The teacher said, "It was as though someone had flicked on a light-switch." She had added, "Joshua is a new boy. He is doing actions in the song time, interacting with the other children, his energy is back, he is not lying around, he is happy!"

His mother told me that Joshua still had much more improving to do in the co-ordination area, but she and her husband would like to say, "How can we thank you enough? You have given us our little boy back!"

Improvements yet to be made now include eye contact and motor co-ordination. I believe that in another 8 months of treatment Joshua will be almost a normal boy.

3 The story of Kirby, who found friends again

A typical ADD/ADHD experience

One of the first children I treated for ADD/ADHD was Kirby, a highly intelligent girl who had become irritable, restless and aggressive around eighteen months of age. Her mother brought her to me at six years and eleven months, despairing at Kirby's hyperactivity, mood swings, irritability, vagueness and poor memory.

Kirby had been considerably affected by her vaccination needles: high temperatures always; at her four-month needle she developed a swollen leg with a hard lump; after her six-month needle she experienced sleeplessness, on-going distress and poor appetite, until a week later when a rash appeared – her immune system firing up. She was soon better, although she remained a restless sleeper.

At nine-and-a-half months, Kirby was given antibiotics, to treat severe nappy rash, and developed thrush. From here on she had many antibiotics – Penicillin, Chloromycetin, Amoxil – all followed by thrush. (This clear sign of *Candida albicans* overload is found in 90% of these children.)

Probably the most unfortunate problem, however, was Kirby's inability to make friends at school. She was too disruptive to be a favourite person to be with! Kirby developed a sugar craving, although she also liked salty foods. Her mother found that chocolate would 'send her off' as did the drug Demazin (for colds), which would take several days to resolve.

Kirby typifies the patients who rapidly respond to our program. When I spoke with her mother ten months later she told me what a changed girl she still is. Now she has some friends and is enrolled in a gifted children's school. She still has to obey the Laws of Health, however and her tendency toward nervousness is still there, but the homoeopathic remedy she takes makes all the difference.

4 The story of Johnny, the providential boy

Johnny was brought to us in 2002. He was eight years old. How he was brought to me is an interesting story.

His mother and father were becoming desperate. They did not want to put him on medication.

One day, his mother was leaving for a journey to Queensland. While waiting for the train, she prayed earnestly that God would lead her to a person who could help Johnny without drugs. Once on the train she sat next to a woman who had boarded from a Sydney station. They got talking, and before long they got to talk about their sons.

When she heard of Johnny's problem, the lady said, "I took my son to Michael Sichel at Fountaindale Clinic in Ourimbah, near Gosford. He really helped more than anybody has been able to before. He specialises in treating ASD children without drugs!"

Some may say that this is coincidence – maybe, and perhaps then we should have renamed our clinic 'The Coincidence Clinic', because I could repeat this providential story from many similar incidents.

Johnny's first appointment was on 20/12/02. Between the age of two and six his parents had seen a decline in his affection and behaviour, plus increasing hyperactivity. His natural immunity had also suffered.

He had been given early antibiotics (end of first year) – in fact, six courses (Amoxil) for 'cellulitis'. (I have noticed 'cellulitis' to be reported post vaccination in several of these children. They were all treated with antibiotics. More on this later.)

His mother reported that Johnny had reactions to later vaccinations, and she refused the last vaccination schedule.

The reactions included:

- Hyperactivity onset
- Affection/eye contact lessened
- School sores were intractable for 12 months (not responding to treatments)
- Allergies began (to food dyes, honey, chocolate, blueberries)

Later, Johnny's attention span at school lessened (ADD), he began to behave impulsively, and became very stubborn.

Significant findings

The boy had gut problems, and what we call 'vascularities' in the liver area (iris reflex). Also, his zinc levels were low; bowels were loose; stool, reported to be unusually smelly; wet his bed until 6 years of age; and had early sugar cravings

His mother had given him a vegetarian diet since weaning (with occasional fish), and identified and removed all known allergic foods and dyes. She had done her best for her child. Without the steps she took, I believe Johnny would have regressed faster, earlier and worse.

Treatment

Johnny was given Metagenics Zinc Drink, digestive enzymes, Blackmore's Bio-C, Natren probiotic bacteria, and Bioceuticals ADFX, a specialist remedy that both calms and increases concentration. It is the herbal equivalent of Ritalin, and works very well, with no side effects (described fully later in book).

He was also prescribed a hearty protein breakfast, a good whole rye bread and protein with salad lunch, and easy to digest food in the evening. And a sugar-free diet.

Outcomes

January 8 – Nineteen days later, his stool was dark and firm. His hyperactivity had lessened. He was happier.

He was given Stevia (from the herb 'sweet leaf') as a sugar replacement, and I asked his mother to test for several foods, including eggs. ('Challenge Test', see pathology chapter).

January 20 – Johnny was on holidays with his parents. They rang in to say, "Johnny is doing very well indeed!"

February 19 – School reports he is 'restless' but his hyperactivity has lessened greatly.

His mother found he reacts to eggs, during the Challenge Test. Eggs had been removed from the diet.

Now I gave Johnny DMG, the natural neuro-transmitter enhancer.

May 8 – Excellent school report. Much improved behaviour, still some hyperactivity, but this seems to be in the normal range for an intelligent active eight year old. However, the improvement has unmasked some early bi-polar symptoms (inclined to be over-excited and later relapse into sadness). This is 'in the family'. Is now using B complex high dose, plus B3 (niacinimide) 800 mg daily, plus magnesium. High doses of these nutrients (higher still for adults and severe bi-polar) will very often clear the problem. One good example: we have an elderly lady client who has been on this program for 34 years. Previous to that she was in mental hospital every Spring, and tried to commit suicide on psyche drugs. She is a normal and highly intelligent lady now – as I said, for 34 years. For her we added ginkgo biloba, which increases circulation to the brain. Once, twenty years ago, thinking she was cured, she ceased the nutrients. The very next week she was in Morrisett Mental Hospital. From there we rescued her and gave her the nutrients. Never again did she go off the program.

These people are poor absorbers. They are not able to take up certain nutrients as another person does. Many mental health cases would be cured if high dose nutrient therapy was carefully applied (see Chapter 9).

5 The story of Jordon

A sad, confused and defiant little boy, who bounced back to 'real' life!

I began to treat Jordon on December 4, 2001. He was possibly the worst Opposition Defiant Disorder (ODD) I had come across.

He had presented 'labelled' as ADHD, with mood swings, aggressive behaviour, extremely hyperactive and unable to concentrate. He was totally 'out-of-control'. As a result he had few or no friends.

He also had trouble getting to sleep and was vague. I found he also had the signs of regressive autism, and had begun to relapse into a shadowy world of his own. At that time, when he was brought to me, he did not know his own name anymore, or his father and mother's name, he did not know which room he slept in and he did not know his sisters' names. He was 'lost' – and his only consolation was watching the dynamic colour and movement of television. He had compulsive obsessive behaviour. For instance, if a cake fell to pieces then he had to try and repair it or have someone else try. Jordon would insist on this, endlessly.

But the worst aspect was his extreme hyperactivity, aggressive and defiant spirit. I remember very well how both Jordon's mother and grandmother (who had come to help control him) were obviously exhausted and at their wits end. They were fit and intelligent women, but with haggard looks and dark eye circles.

December 5, 2001 – Mother phoned me. She acted on my advice and giving him the natural remedies I prescribed. **Within 24 hours his mother reported, "I can't believe the change so quick! He woke up quietly for the first time in ages and peacefully ate the protein breakfast you suggested – no anger, no fuss."**

Following this, there were several follow-up conversations, and one visit.

March 12, 2002 – Mother and grandmother reported: socializing better; 35% language improvement; bowels now OK (had been very loose); attention improved; eating much better.

March 5, 2003 – One year later, they visited me again. Jordon is now 4 yrs old. **I could hardly recognise him as the same boy! He had improved so much. He was now a delightful little boy, obedient, loving and even thoughtful.** He still has occasional mood swings, but so do many normal boys. His speech was almost normal.

His treatment is ongoing for another year. He could easily regress if the treatment is not continued until his physiology is completely repaired. This restoration has been the result of dietary changes and times of eating plus the administration of the repair nutrients and neuro-transmitter enhancers.

This had been a wonderful turn-around.

There are many stories like these on our records. More than 85% of our Alphabet kids come good or improve significantly. Usually the hyperactive component goes within 4 days! You will read 'why' and 'how' later in this book.

But not only do we have Alphabet Kids, we also have Alphabet Adults who have come good. And many young teenagers.

Let me share with you the story of 23-year old Ken.

6 The 'ADHD' electrician who nearly lost his job

Ken came to us from Sydney. He was holding down a good job in his trade. But he was an 'Alphabet' man. For several years he had fought the demon of ADHD. It was the hyperactivity component that was threatening his job.

I changed his meal times around, so he ate his major meal for breakfast, with emphasis on protein. This enabled him to easily endure the removal of sugar from his diet (see the Nutritional section for full explanation of this important step).

He was taken off all sugars, including fruit and juices, and his milk products.

He was given Horopito herb for his *candidiasis* (yeast infection), bacteria for his bowels, and digestive enzymes.

At the end of the first week on this program he called from Sydney and said to me that his hyperactivity was no longer present. Moreover, he was thinking clearly again and his work was not in jeopardy anymore! He said, "I am so grateful to you!"

Ken was one of many hundreds of adults with 'altered minds' who we have reversed by using functional medicine methods to treat the intestinal system and bloodstream.

7 Joe, the 12-year old low IQ ADD boy who reached his potential

Joe came with his mother in 2000. They lived on a farm, surrounded by fresh mountain air and peace. But Joe had developed a certain 'slowness' around 3 years of age. This 'slowness' of thought and normal progression in skills, language and later, particularly reading – caused his parents concern.

Now he was 12 years of age, and at the bottom of his class. He just could not read very well at all, he could not learn and life was becoming a burden for him.

When he presented, he looked very depressed, uptight and most unhappy. His mother was deeply concerned for him. He had been diagnosed and his 'Alphabet' was ADD.

His IQ had been measured and was below normal.

Treatment

After the usual dietary changes, I used every neuro-transmitter (NT) remedy available, one by one. And then in combination. First testing him for zinc. But zinc was normal.

We began with the amino-acid L. glutamine. He was given 3,000 mg twice daily.

On the next appointment, one month later, Joe was quite excited. His teacher had found that Joe had stepped up a level in his reading.

He was then given another NT to add to the glutamine, plus the Bioceutical ADFX. He kept this up for three months, and then came to see me with his mother.

This time Joe was positively beaming! He was happy and relaxed. He had jumped upward through the class and was now nearly in the middle, average! He was playing sport again (his former depression had made him lose interest).

Best of all, his mother told me that he now had hopes of a future job. He didn't aim high for that, just a job. He knew his potential had been reached, at least for his age. Maybe that potential would increase as he matured. "Late starters are often the most successful in the end," I said to his mother and him. And he came from a hard working and successful Greek background.

8 The Aspergers boy who changed in two days on diet alone!

This story from England, illustrates the work now proceeding around the world

When this little boy was born, he was immediately put on antibiotics to 'protect him from a virus' (his parents were told). This commenced a downward trend in his health. As he grew his ill health continued. While a baby, he was always vomiting and picked up every infection around.

As is almost universal in ASD problems, his sleeping patterns were abnormal. For the first two years of his life, he would only sleep for two or three minutes at a time before waking. When he reached the age of three, this pattern reversed and he began sleeping excessively in the afternoons. As he grew older his parents began to notice unusual behaviours. He did not seem to be like other children.

The most distinctive sign was that when excited or was concentrating on something, he would flap his arms quickly. Tom also became vacant at times, disappearing into a world of his own. He also began shaking involuntarily and had terrible temper tantrums over things that other children would not react to.

His mother was convinced that something was wrong.

A teacher at nursery school who had worked with autistic children, suggested that Tom be taken to the family doctor for a test. The doctor referred them to a specialist who assessed Tom as suffering from Asperger Syndrome.

Tom was then taken to a doctor at the local hospital who specialised in treating ASD problems with dietary changes. This doctor used the same urine tests to measure the permeability of the small intestine, as we do in Australia (see Pathology Chapter).

Briefly, the intestinal permeability (IP) test tells whether a child is "leaking" larger than normal food molecules through his gut walls. Certain proteins (milk casein and grain gluten) can thus enter the bloodstream. Once there, some particles reach the brain and act on the brain with a morphine-like affect. (For this reason they are called casomorphine and glutomorphine).

Because Tom had been given antibiotics almost continuously for the first six months of his life, the doctor knew that his gut would have been disrupted in this manner. Urine tests confirmed that he had high levels of peptide (food)-morphines in his blood.

So, Tom commenced the gluten-free, dairy-free diet. He was also taken off sugars, which can also affect the brain.

Changes in two days!

His parents noticed a difference after just two days on the diet.

"It was really dramatic," said his mother. "Normally on long car journeys Tom and I would sit in silence as he was absorbed in his own world. But this time we were driving and he said 'Look Mummy, there's a cow' and I almost crashed the car! It was the first time he has ever taken an interest in his surroundings like that."

In just four months, his mother has been astounded by the change in his behaviour.

She said he is becoming generally more aware of what is going on around him and has started taking an interest in other people – such as by asking them questions. He has also started remembering more information and can recall it more easily than before.

Another sign which is common to Alphabet Children are dark circles under the eyes, caused by allergies. Tom also suffered from these circles but since starting the diet, they have virtually disappeared.

The biggest change in Tom's behaviour was his interaction with other children. His mother noticed that before starting the diet Tom wouldn't join in the conversations other children would be having. He was always too involved in his own busy activities, such as obsessively lining up all his toys in neat rows. He never used to have one special friend but now has a big group of friends. His condition has improved so much that there is now hope that he may one day completely recover.

NOTE: In my own practice I would endeavour to further improve Tom by use of bacteria/probiotics (bowel flora), nutrient powders that repair the gut, digestive enzymes to improve the digestion, natural medicines that increase the stomach enzyme production plus natural neuro-transmitter enhancers for the brain. (See: Treatments Chapter).

9 Two regressive Autism boys

Regressive autism occurs when a normally developing child begins to lose learned behaviours and skills. These may include losing some words or all speech, loss of affection, eye contact, motor co-ordination, reading ability, social skills, etc. Sometimes, unusual skills will develop in some area (maybe maths or puzzles), plus often compulsive unusual behaviour appears. This may include what is called 'stimming' (self hurting, head banging, or spinning on the spot). But each child is different. These changes usually occur around 2½–3 years of age.

These two stories are short, but are intended to show how quickly even this terrifying disease can be reversed ('terrifying' for the parents). Because the reversal of such a disease takes time, any improvement is welcomed. These improvements usually occur one at a time. That autism is curable is proved by at least eight sets of parents who have written a book on their child's deliverance.

Dan, a boy with Regressive Autism/Global Developmental Delay (GDD)

This diagnosis was given at the Westmead Children's Hospital in 2002. The word regressive means that not only does a child not advance, but actually goes backward.

This type of autism (which accounts for probably 90% of all autism in Australia – and rising) points to some disease process that usually manifests at 2½–3 years of age. This is now affecting tens of thousands of children world-wide with regular frequency about one year after they receive a raft of twenty-four immunisation vaccines (by eighteen months).

Strong scientific evidence now confirms a probable autoimmune reaction to the measles vaccine component in autism spectrum disorders. This evidence, published in April 2003, was a controlled study and the reaction was found in 83% of autistic children, but not in normal children, nor the healthy twin of autistic siblings. (Singh & Jensen, Utah University). This study was the latest in a long line of evidence from several respected Universities (including Harvard) that began in 1998, where measles vaccine virus has been found in gut, brain and spinal cord tissues.

The causal relationship to autism has been denied from the start by the orthodox establishment and Governments. Does that sound familiar? This maybe one reason why the term regressive autism appears to be changing to 'global developmental delay'. GDD puts the blame on the child – he is delayed, abnormally stupid or disordered. Whereas, 'regressive' means he was normal, but suddenly (not long after the triple-antigen DTP vaccination – often implicated in strong reactions) he begins to lose the gains his quest for life had won for him.

In Dan's case, the first backward steps began when he was 2½ years. By 5½ years of age he had lost all speech. He could no longer say numbers, which he had begun to learn. He began to bang his head against walls and chairs, he became disruptive and anti-social. He had aversion to the colour red. He found revulsion to the feel of certain clothes. His bowels were disrupted, and alternating between hard and soft. They were abnormally potent with smell. He became terribly excited by the vacuum cleaner.

When the parents brought him to me he was unhappy and restless. His hyperactivity plainly upset his parents, who were managing him well but very tired. This was because he woke through the night – several times and every night. Both parents worked.

I spent two hours with them and explained what had happened to their boy and how we were going to reverse at least some of his problems. When they left, they were convinced this was the way to go and determined to implement the advice.

Two weeks later, I saw them again. Dan's hyperactivity was obviously far less, and his parents confirmed that. They said he was more settled, and his bowels had improved after only seven days. His sleep was better, but still disturbing early in the morning hours. He still had no words, but his response to his parents had improved noticeably.

These improvements came about with the usual low allergy diet, plus being gluten-casein-sugar-and-chocolate-free. He had been given a selenium sub-lingual spray. (Selenium is a potent anti-oxidant which in controlled trials, has been shown to reduce allergies of all types significantly.) He also had been given liquid zinc, and dimethylglycine (DMG). I further ordered a gastro-intestinal permeability test.

This second visit, I added essential fatty acids, magnesium, digestive enzymes and *Bifidobacterium infantis* probiotics.

One week later, Dan came back again. **His parents told me he had begun saying words again!** He had picked up the telephone and spoken into it (copying his parents) and was sleeping all night. He had also lost his dislike of the colour red.

These were all significant changes. **The total changes had taken only three weeks**!

But Dan, as of this writing, is still much delayed in speech and I advised the parents to seek a skilled practitioner in speech therapy. Now that his internal chaos is largely clear, and his behaviour is more normal and he is a happier boy, speech therapy will have a much better possibility of early and good success.

Trent, another boy with Regressive Autism

This 7-year old came at end of February, 2003. He had also been diagnosed with Global Developmental Delay. He had also lost speech and communication abilities. This had begun to be noticed at 3–3½ years.

His parents appeared to be determined to follow the drug-free program, but the father later admitted he was very sceptical.

The first few weeks commenced with the usual GF-CF-SF diet. He was given *Bifidobacterium infantis* and homeopathic drops under the tongue to counteract possible excessive cortico steroid involvement. This was because his mother had a problem with over active adrenal production during pregnancy (Cushings Syndrome).

I ordered an Intestinal Permeability Test. This came back positive – he had a 'leaky gut', as most of these children do (Dr Tim Buie, Harvard Med. School, 2002).

I also ordered a Complete Digestive Stool Analysis, which showed digestive dysfunction – especially with handling of fatty acids (a common problem with these children).

But in less than 10 days his family noticed positive changes. He began to share things, slept more and was more affectionate.

After these results came back, I added digestive enzymes, essential fatty acids and additional gastric enzyme support.

By the beginning of June, the changes had been very encouraging. His sister reported that he was now playful, much more alert and 'alive'. He was also positively affectionate.

Now we commenced vitamin B6 in high doses along with magnesium. And also added DMG, to be taken two weeks after the experiment with the B6 and magnesium (this is a standard therapy for autism).

The father noted that even more positive 'brain' events began to happen, especially after the DMG. (This reflects the excellent results obtained by the American Autism Research Institute with DMG – 42% of 4,725 children got better).

So, in a few weeks this boy was literally coming alive again.

Long-term therapy

More total repair of these serious cases will take time. However, as long as there has been no damage in the womb or at birth then we expect to see dramatic improvements.

The one uncertain factor, for me, is the long-term damage done by the mercury and other known poisons and neuro-toxins used in the vaccines.

Fortunately, the public outcry against mercury in particular has forced even the Governments and pharma-cartels to partly remove or lower the amount of this very potent toxin (but not until around 2001). However, it is still used in some vaccines. There is still a long way to go – they still use aluminium, anti-freeze, formaldehyde and many other excipients, and antibiotic preservatives (depending on the vaccine).

The single most important lesson from this Chapter

Your child's immune system is the hero ...

Bearing in mind that functional medicine achieves its results by aiding the child's total body well-being return to normal function, how can such widespread gains be accredited to such simple remedies and life-style changes? The simple answer – it can't be.

Widespread gains of this magnitude cannot be due to any single 'magic bullet'. That credit is not due to the remedies and methods we use, but to their total combined effects in normalising and unleashing the great power inherent in the immune system of your child.

Therefore, in my opinion and that of many others, Immune System Functional Improvement (ISFI) should be the major focus of the scientific community involved in the current childhood epidemic.

Let me illustrate the latent power of an immune system freed, even partially, from the burdens of nutritional deficiencies, toxic overloads, 'germs', yeasts, heavy metals and vaccination effects. **Even cancers have been cured by immune system improvement**.

> 'The indisputable fact that tumours may spontaneously regress provides the basic incentive to develop biological and specific immunological cancer therapies. This implies that mammals possess a natural intrinsic regulatory capability to control the differentiation of specialized organ cells. Dietary correction of the aetiological metabolic deficiency, supported by autologous

(meaning inherent to the patient) active specific immunotherapy in patients suffering from metastatic renal adenocarcinoma, or malignant melanoma, have caused highly significant clinical results, as compared with our best standard therapies, in randomised clinical series which comprised hundreds of patients, with a follow-up over thirty years.

Initially hard to explain, the therapeutic result was a complete disappearance of large tumours.'

Development of Combined Biological & Immunological Cancer Therapy Modality. A review of bio-immunotherapy.Thomas Tallberg, Dr Med)

The full article appeared in the Journal of the Australasian College of Nutritional and Environmental Medicine, Vol. 22, No. 1, April 2003, pages 3–21. It can be viewed at www.acnem.org. ACNEM is the College of the medical community in Australasia which specialise in natural medicine and immune system enhancement.

Now, the question has to be asked: if such a deadly and complex disease as cancer can be cured by the power of an 'educated' immune system, then what can this same immune system do to make common children's infections (measles, mumps, whooping cough, chicken pox, etc) a 'normal' part of growing-up? As they once used to be. For once a child has been exposed to a 'wild' strain (natural infection), they are immune for life. But not so with immunisation (and often not even immune at all). Some may say, 'but cancer cells are abnormal and it is a chronic disease, not an infectious entity'. And the simple answer to that is: if immune systems are NOT able to control infections like flu, SARS, measles, mumps, etc. then why don't ALL children and adults get the infection when exposed to it? Because many don't!"

This immune system approach is being seen by many parents around the world as a true answer to ASD. Here is a typical letter, from a German parent who once worked in the pharmaceutical industry.

"The research for a curable treatment of this disease goes totally in the wrong direction, as pharmaceutical drugs are researched, or drugs for a neurological disease are tested. This disease is an autoimmune disease and in the first place a gastrointestinal problem affecting the brain as the children's brain are starving essential nutrients as their digestive systems are damaged and not functioning properly. The children have a chance to recover if the right doctors will understand the link between heavy metals and the gut/brain connection. This disease can only be cured with biomedical interventions and a total turn in lifestyle (American diet, nutrition environmental thinking etc.). Sometimes I think those children are messengers to tell us: Stop with all this pollution, toxins etc. We have broken the laws of nature incredibly and we can only fix it with natural approaches and perhaps the society – not only in the USA but everywhere – have to make a big turn that our people stay healthy in this very toxic world. My very best and thank you for all this efforts."

Bettina Metz, mother of an 7-year old autistic boy

CHAPTER SIX

Pathology

Specialist ASD pathology

Helps us diagnose your child's internal environment, plus major deficiencies, toxic metals & chemicals

In tandem with the growing knowledge of the gut/brain connection and the other major environmental problems that cause learning and behavioural problems, new methods of pathology have lately been developed. These both confirm the functional causative theory and aid in diagnosis and tracking of treatments. Some of these methods have been around for many years (as hair tissue mineral assays – or 'hair analysis'), but often prove themselves indispensable in ASD problems. Between them, these very useful pathology results can tell us exactly what your child is lacking, or is overloaded with in the matter of nutrients and toxic substances such as mercury, lead etc, together with digestive function tests. Any significant discrepancies must be dealt with before other therapies can work.

The following abnormal nutrient profile is common in ASD's:

> Low in vitamins A, B6, B12, C, D and E, and in Omega-6 essential fatty acids (EFA's), zinc, magnesium and selenium. Also, reduced sulphates are available for essential detoxification procedures in liver functions. This is the mechanism that can malfunction if sufficient sulphur is not available and makes many ASD's sensitive to the phenols contained in apples, oranges, bananas, grapes, chocolate, food colourings and some herbs and spices. (So far, no child has been found deficient in Ritalin!) Several amino acids are consistently low in ASD's. Digestive enzymes are also found to be deficient in these children.

Other pathologies can specifically tell us the efficiency of the digestive system itself. Others identify levels of gastro-intestinal inhabitants (both friendly and pathogenic), such as *E. coli, streptoccus* (common in ASD), *staph, amoeba,* parasites and fungal pathogens like *Candida albicans* and *Candida glabrata* (also common in ASD).

Digestive function & gut environment testing

These internal environment and function tests are also very important, because they can tell us, objectively, if your child has a 'leaky' gut, leading to the malabsorption that causes the multiple nutrient deficiencies above plus cognitive disorders.

These tests are made possible by placing stool or urine samples in small containers (supplied by the laboratory). The lab can then perform a number of revealing tests.

It is now well established that most ASD children have intestinal problems. In my 57 children study group, 84% reported digestive/gut symptoms. This reflects the findings now recorded around the world.

The hormone secretin is used by some practitioners to increase the release of pancreatic enzymes, so vital in digestion. Secretin is released when sufficient acidity is sensed by the secretor in the duodenum. This then becomes the hormonal signal for the pancreas activity, and begins a stream of 'spurts' of digestive enzymes (as proteinase, lipase, etc) into the partially digested food from the stomach.

However, in our clinic we prefer to begin the treatment at the source of this digestive cascade, which is the stomach. The children who have these problems, and many do, are not producing sufficient stomach acids to trigger the hormone secretin. By using stomach remedies, we endeavour to stimulate the natural acid production.

Immune system tests

Other tests can tell us of your child's ability to detoxify the body via the liver. Efficient liver function is necessary for the processing and excretion of drugs, hormones and chemicals.

Heavy metal testing

Two examples of severe effects in children

Testing is also available for the damaging metals like mercury, cadmium, arsenic, aluminium and lead levels (blood, urine or hair analysis), as well as the necessary vitamin/mineral levels.

I have found them very useful. For instance, while writing this new edition one of our clients, a ten year old boy with intractable learning problems, was brought to me for treatment. He was placed on the usual clear-and-restore program, and responded quite fast but not satisfactorily. He was a bright boy, keen to do well, but just couldn't concentrate or learn. His mind was sluggish.

I questioned his mother and found his years from birth until nine had been spent living near a large plastics manufacturing factory. The house was also on a busy main road, and both mother and son remembered the exhaust fumes flooding the home.

I then suggested we perform a hair tissue mineral analysis for both nutrient and toxic metals (nutrients like calcium, magnesium, zinc and also bad metals like lead, mercury and cadmium etc). When this came back we found elevated lead, cadmium and aluminium levels. Lead's role in learning difficulties is well-known.

The next task was to chelate metals (chelation, from the Greek word *chele*, 'to claw out'). I sent him to a medical centre which specialises in chelation.

The lead girl

Paranoia & uncontrollable raging tantrums from toxic metal

More recently, an apparently intractable seven year old girl was brought to me. Deeply disturbed, she clung to her mother in fear – yet attacked her and her sister at other times, with real anger – biting, kicking and hitting. Her sister was brave to the constant ordeals, but it was taking its toll. The girl also had phobias, and was deeply fearful of making decisions or any change in routines. A psychiatrist could not give any specific diagnosis, despite several expensive visits. The only clue was an exposure to lead-laden dust that lasted for several days when younger. But later blood tests showed no contamination. Nevertheless, because I knew that after the initial exposure period has passed, blood is a poor recorder of heavy metals, I ordered a hair analysis. I also ordered the digestive and gut permeability tests.

Meanwhile, while waiting for the tests, she was given several relevant biological remedies. These brought little change, although some improvement after two weeks of applying an ayurvedic calming oil to her skin nightly.

When the hair analysis arrived it showed the highest lead level I had ever seen – three times higher than the 'normal' or average expected range. (Although a true 'normal' to me would be 'zero'). This was a confirmation to me of the uselessness of blood lead testing sometime well after an exposure to lead. The body buffers the blood and quickly shunts toxins like lead into 'safer' places in the body – often into fat, or other cells where least harm can occur.

Individual reactions to toxin exposure – chaos to calm

In looking through the literature on the effects of lead on various individuals I came across the case of a physician who became mentally ill with a diagnosis of paranoid schizophrenia. "Ah!" I thought, "Here is a parallel example to this little girl."

But with one major difference, the physician was a fully grown man of thirty-three years. His hair analysis showed lead four times greater than 'normal', but his body mass was much greater than my little patient, and thus able to handle such a load a little better.

The physician had taken to alcohol and psychoactive drugs to control his problem. Following chelation therapy (intravenous amino acid drips that 'claw' out heavy metals) he had returned to normal and no longer craved alcohol or drugs.

Now the girl is having her chelation therapy and she is improving.

Arsenic

I am finding that arsenic is also a problem among my child clients. This has not been highlighted before to the extent of mercury and lead, but is showing up among my client population as a single cause of behavioural problems in several recent cases.

A recent study found six out of ten ASD behaviourally damaged children had high levels of arsenic compared to NIL among a control group of healthy children. Lately, too, the use of arsenic in wood preservation is, I understand, being discontinued. Timber preserved this way is found in fences and constructions around both homes and schools.

Arsenic is included in several categories of psychiatric problems caused by heavy metals, below.

The many ways in which toxic metals can affect your child

Psychiatric disturbances

Social Deficits, Social withdrawal
Mercury

Repetitive, perseverative, stereotyped behaviours; OCD-typical behaviors
Mercury

Depression, mood swings, flat affect; impaired facial recognition
Arsenic, Copper, Lead, Mercury

Schizoid tendencies; hallucinations; delirium
Mercury

Irritability, aggressive behaviors, temper tantrums
Lead, Mercury

Suicidal Behaviors
Copper, Mercury

Sleep difficulties/ disturbances
Lead, Mercury, Thallium

Chronic fatigue (CFS); weakness, malaise
Aluminium, Arsenic, Cadmium, Copper, Lead, Mercury, Thallium

Anorexia; symptoms reflecting eating disorders, loss of appetite/weight
Arsenic, Lead, Mercury

Anxiety; nervous tendencies
Thallium

Attention problems (ADHD), lacks eye contact, impaired visual fixation
Lead, Mercury

Speech and language deficits

Speech disorders
Aluminium, Mercury

Loss of speech, developmental problems with language
Mercury

Speech comprehension deficits
Mercury

Dysarthria; articulation problems; slurred speech, unintelligible speech
Mercury

Cognitive impairments

Mental retardation, borderline intelligence
Arsenic, Lead, Mercury

Uneven performance on IQ scores, low IQ scores
Copper, Lead

Poor concentration, attention deficits (ADHD), response inhibition
Aluminium, Lead

Poor memory (short term, verbal, and auditory)
Aluminium, Lead

Difficulties understanding abstract ideas; difficulty carrying out complex commands
X metals

Dementia; pre-senile and senile dementia
Aluminum

Stupor
Aluminum, Arsenic,

Impaired reaction time; lower performance on timed tests
Lead

Sensory abnormalities

Abnormal Sensations in the mouth and extremities
Arsenic

Hearing loss, difficulty hearing
Arsenic, Lead, Mercury

Abnormal touch sensations; diminished touch sensations, aversion to touch
Arsenic

Blurred vision; sensitivity to light
Arsenic, Mercury

Motor disorders

Choreiform movements, myoclonal jerks, unusual postures
Copper, Mercury

Difficulty walking, swallowing, talking
Copper, Mercury

Flapping, circling, rocking, toe walking
Mercury

Problems with intentional movements or imitation
Mercury

Abnormal gait/posture; incoordination, loss of balance; problems sitting, lying, crawling, and walking
Mercury

Decreased locomotor activity
Aluminum, Arsenic

Convulsions; seizure
Aluminum, Arsenic, Copper, Lead, Mercury, Thallium

Physiological impairment

Brain and Central Nervous System

Neurofibrillary tangles
Aluminum

Neuritis, retrobulbar neuritis; neuropathy
Aluminum, Arsenic, Thallium

Encephalopathy
Aluminum, Arsenic, Lead, Thallium

Cerebrovascular disease
X metals

Alterations in nerve conduction velocity
Lead

Alterations in the spinal chord
Thallium

Accumulates in CNS structures
Aluminum, Mercury

Abnormal EEGs
Arsenic, Lead

Autonomic disturbances
Copper, Lead, Mercury, Thallium

Peripheral Nervous System

Peripheral neuropathy
Arsenic, Mercury

Alterations in peripheral nerves
Arsenic

Loss of feeling/ numbness in the extremities; paresthesia
Arsenic, Mercury, Thallium

Gastrointestinal Tract

Nausea, vomiting, diarrhea; loss of appetite
Arsenic, Copper, Mercury, Thallium

Abdominal pain, stomach cramps; burning of the throat and mouth
Arsenic, Copper, Lead, Mercury, Thallium

Esophagitis; gastroenteritis; colitis
Arsenic, Mercury, Thallium

Cancers (colon, pancreatic, stomach, or rectal)
Arsenic

Renal and hepatic impairment

Hepatotoxicity; Liver dysfunction, damage
Arsenic, Copper, Thallium

Cirrhosis of the liver; hepatitis
Copper

Kidney disease ; kidney failure
Arsenic, Lead, Mercury

Renal toxicity; tubular proteinosis
Arsenic, Copper, Lead

Kidney Damage, histological alterations
Arsenic, Lead

Cardiovascular System

Blood vessel damage
Arsenic

Anemia; decreased red blood cell count
Arsenic, Copper, Lead

Hypertension; increased heart rate (tachycardia)
Arsenic, Copper, Lead, Thallium

Electrocardiac disorders

Peripheral vascular disease; cardiovascular disease; vascular collapse
Arsenic, Lead

Respiratory System

Pulmonary Fibrosis
Aluminum, Arsenic

Pulmonary edema
X metals

Pneumonia, laryngitis, pharyngitis, bronchitis
Aluminum, Arsenic, Mercury

Restrictive airway disorders, asthmatic conditions, pneumoconiosis
Arsenic, Aluminum

Respiratory tract cancers
Arsenic

Nasal ulcers, perforation of the nasal septum
X metals

Immune System

Increased incidences of asthma, autoimmune-like symptoms, & allergies
X metals

Inhibition of lymphocytes, T-cells, monocytes
X metals

Immunosuppression
Lead

Decreased white blood cell count
Arsenic, Thallium

Reproductive System

Genital abnormalities
Aluminum, Thallium

Disturbances in menstrual cycle; menstrual pains
Copper, Mercury

Birth defects; premature births; Spontaneous abortion
Arsenic, Lead, Mercury

Reproductive dysfunction
Arsenic, Aluminum, Cadmium, Lead

Other Physical Disturbances

Hypotonia or hypertonia; decreased muscular strength
X metals

Rashes, contact dermatitis, eczema, itchy/irritating skin
Aluminum, Arsenic, Copper, Mercury

Muscle pain; headache; acrodynia; colic
Arsenic, Copper, Lead, Thallium

Alopecia (hair loss)
Thallium

Even low-level exposure to chemicals and heavy metals can have a powerful impact on the human body. Autoimmune diseases (such as lupus and multiple sclerosis), Parkinson's-like symptoms, chronic fatigue syndrome and ***cardiovascular disease*** are common responses to toxic chemicals and heavy metals – but they aren't the only ones. Memory loss, lower IQ's, increased allergic reactions, high blood pressure and failing immune systems also result from these exposures.

Chelation therapy is a safe, non-surgical treatment used to rid the body of excess toxins, particularly metals. These chelators have the ability to draw out toxic metals and other harmful substances that impair bodily functions and help the body eliminate these toxins via the kidneys. Oral Chelating agents can often prevent health problems from occurring by restoring circulation to the body's tissues. Chelation benefits every blood vessel in the body, from the largest veins to the tiniest capillaries and arterioles, most of which are too small for surgical treatment or too deep within the brain and other vital organs to be safely reached by surgery.

We would like to thank *Extreme Health*, www.autismmercury.com, for providing this highly referenced chart on how the many ways toxic heavy metals have the ability to affect the body. Extreme Health provides an Oral Chelation Formula, which has been used with great success on children diagnosed with autism, aspergers, ADHD etc. You may read detailed success stories written by parents on their web site. I thoroughly recommend a look on this site.

Organic acid testing

Test are also available for Organic Acids. The relative balance of fatty acids and others tell us a great deal about digestive function. Microbial panels, Gluten/Casein sensitivity, and amino tests and peptides, plus Basic Food Allergy – Inhalant Allergies, all add to the picture when necessary.

Definitive and low cost test for *candidiasis*

The Spit Test

First thing in the morning, before you put anything in your child's mouth, fill a clear glass with pure or filtered water. Now, have your child work up some saliva, and then spit it into the water. For the next hour, check the water about every 15 minutes. If there is a candida yeast infection, you will see strings traveling down into the water from the saliva floating on the top, or 'cloudy' saliva will sink to the bottom of the glass, or cloudy specks will be seen to be suspended in the water. If nothing develops in that hour, your child is probably candida free.

If you think there is evidence, then the next step is to positively identify and quantify the infection. Abnormal candida yeast levels have always been difficult to ascertain and follow-up, unless costly testing was used. But since March 2003, a laboratory (Australian Biologics, Sydney, Ph 02 9283 0807) has introduced a new low-cost test that is simple to use. This is another pathology for which many practitioners are very thankful. The Enzyme-Linked Immunosorbent Assay (ELISA) allows us to know with certainty, if an abnormal level of *Candida* is playing a part in your child's ASD problems.

Testing for allergies

Accompanying ASDs, ADD/HD

Three allergy tests we use in our clinic are:

- ***Challenge testing.*** This is the simplest and most accurate, in our experience. It can be combined with the Pulse Test. It is a home test, and costs nothing!
  To 'challenge' a food: leave that particular food from the diet for five days. On the sixth day, serve a considerable serving at breakfast (however, if a serious allergy is suspected see a practitioner with knowledge in this field).
- ***Cytotoxic testing.*** The laboratory testing of a blood sample for metabolic intolerance, which is about 70% accurate.

- *Pulse testing.* Compares the pulse rates on waking (basal pulse – the lowest pulse of the day), the resting pulse before each meal, and at three half-hourly intervals after each meal. Wide variations are evidence of some allergic reaction to foods eaten at the previous meal.

Generally, we do not consider allergy testing until the underlying problems are at least partly resolved. The major allergens/sensitivities are usually recognised by the mothers before they come to us. We encourage them to continue in their efforts to remove these known items.

The reason for this methodology is that the average child who presents is probably more or less sensitive to 50% or more of what he eats and will continue to be until the gut and digestion are improved. But gut and digestion can be improved quite rapidly, and when the signs of such improvement are obvious, then one or another method of testing can be arranged. Improving signs include normal bowel movements, less or nil stomach/gut pains and bloating, better sleep, less general feeling of malaise (tired, sick-feeling, feeling 'yucky') and significant lessening of flatulence (or crepitus, as medicine politely names it). Always a welcome change for the family!

More objective and accurate estimation of such improvement is now possible through the use of repeated digestive and leaky-gut pathology.

But allergies can certainly be the single cause of many unusual symptoms. Here are two examples:

Case history 1 – the violent boy

A hyperactive thirteen-year-old was brought to us by his mother, a nurse, because of his violent and aggressive behaviour. He was found to have thirty-six allergic reactions out of a possible seventy. Several of these were severe and, typical of many allergy victims, almost all of them related to foods that he commonly ate, and in the greatest quantity.

Substituting the chief culprit foods and helping the gut to repair calmed him down.

Case history 2 – the sneezing boy

One five-and-a-half-year-old boy was brought to me because of a serious and chronic sneezing problem. His nurse mother said he had been sneezing on and off for five years, sometimes sneezing a hundred times without stopping, and his mother had been unable to find help anywhere. She was naturally sceptical when, after examining his diet, and asking a few pertinent questions about the boy's bowel habits, it was possible to establish that the boy had an allergy to milk, wheat and oranges. With a change in the boy's eating habits and the aid of some digestive enzyme tablets, his sneezing problem left in two days – permanently.

Improving digestion

We have said a lot about the effects of foods on health and suggested that improving digestion and later taking away the allergens may help many health problems, including autism spectrum disorders, ADD and ADHD.

Bio-individuality is a major factor in prescribing a course of treatment for malfunctioning digestion. And while an experienced practitioner can improve an individual's digestive processes, there are many variables to consider. Some patients, we find, have under-active stomachs, others have a lack of bile production, and many have a number of causes.

And these problems are in no way restricted to children.

Fortunately there are many very effective remedies for improving the various digestive malfunctions. These include:

- Supplying the missing enzymes in tablet form;
- Stimulating the glands themselves to work more productively;
- Soothing & repairing the often inflamed & damaged mucosa of the intestine;
- Replacing the vital intestinal flora;
- Altering the pH (acid/alkaline balance) of the large bowel and the stomach; and
- Adding vital nutrients that rebuild the walls and other tissue connected with the gastrointestinal tract.

Improving the 'internal environment' as outlined in this book, is the single most important measure we take to restore damaged children (and adults). And we have been applying that principle, with growing knowledge, for 40 years!

CHAPTER SEVEN

Alkalizing and balancing the Alphabet Kids

Dealing with the mercury and other heavy metals

To successfully treat ASD children, with or without heavy metal problems, it is absolutely essential to maintain an average body pH that is alkaline – not acid. Only in that range can the body function properly. Also, that alkaline range is required to get rid of toxic metals like mercury, lead, arsenic, antimony and cadmium (a process known as 'chelation'). Taking any form of Chelation without attending to this factor will be very inefficient, if not impossible.

It is very important for you to understand the significance of this procedure, then – in my experience with many families, you will take this step seriously. It needs to be taken seriously, as it is the single most important easily changed physical condition in your child's body.

This is because our bodies are like a high-functioning factory of continuous and rapid chemical reactions that are essential to life. This amazing chemical activity could never be reproduced artificially at such high speed. The activity mostly takes place in and around our cells. New research has found that the cell walls are not really 'walls' at all, but rather like a fluctuating liquid frontier allowing 'business transactions across the border' all aimed at maintaining a **balance** for maximum efficiency. **Our children have lost their balance.**

This balance is significantly upset by 'heavy metals' like mercury, lead and arsenic, commonly found in ASD children. These alter the balance of the **essential** metals – like calcium, magnesium, zinc and more than 60 others, and can produce many symptoms. The heavy metals are also toxic in themselves.

One of the most important 'balancing acts' is the acid/alkaline ratio in both the internal environment of the cell itself and the surrounding gel-like fluid in which the cells live. This acid/alkaline ratio is called the pH. **A correct pH is vital to good health and function.** It is a mechanism with many implications.

Your child's average body fluid pH can easily be measured by a urine test at home. The best range is 7.3 for females and 7.6 for males. Anything below 6.9 is not good.

Most of the children we measure have a 4.6 to 6.3 reading, which is far too acid.

Just like any factory, a child's body produces wastes that can become toxic to the body if they are not eliminated. The body factory uses the bloodstream to carry wastes along the factory 'pipeline' blood vessels to the liver and kidneys, for final disposal. These wastes include all kinds of toxins and excesses plus poisons produced by enemy pathogens (exotoxins, endotoxins, mycotoxins). This is why we ask the question: "How often does your child go to the toilet?". Some children do not move their bowels more than three times a week... but eat three times daily! You can imagine the plumbing 'log-jamb' and toxins being released. This is one major factor that leads to acidity. Acidity is the enemy of good health – and the ally of inflammatory conditions, including cancer.

This acidity occurs because the toxins have the total affect of lowering the urine to a minus or 'negative' pH. Some foods also do this if eaten in excess. (See list below). Unfortunately, if a body has a low pH the heavy metals remain 'electrically charged'. They then behave like the static electricity which causes nylon to stick to wool' and they 'stick' to the tissues in your child's body, making it impossible to easily rid itself of these potent nerve toxins. This was discovered over one hundred years ago, by an English scientist called H.J. Fenton - in 1894.

Recently, we have seen some amazing changes in both children and adults by simply applying this natural law and maintaining their body pH optiminally (one adult client phoned me this morning and said: "You have saved my life". He had been very ill for years and worsening. That is another story).

One of these clients was a lady who had successfully fought leukemia (CLL) for eight years, without having to use chemotherapy. She had been the amazement of her oncologist, and learned how to help herself through a world-wide net of other CLL victims. But in the last two years her white cell count had begun to rise out-of-control. She had begun to feel tired and in pain. We had helped her with her nutritional program and suggested she may like to raise her pH to a safer level (it was very acid). The response came almost immediately, with total pain relief in two days. She bought an electronic pH meter to improve both monitoring and accuracy.

She has continued on this for three months and still has no pain. Her regular visits to the oncologist also shows improvement in the health of the white cells (they are less cancerous). She has other CLL friends around the world using this health improving method, all finding similar results.

In one family, with twin ASD boys, the child not responding so well 'turned the corner' within 12 hours of commencement of his alkalizing program. He began to forge ahead and passed his brother in language and reading skills for the first time. This was after three years of treatments, which had improved them both (but one, as I said, more than the other). That twin had been first in line for receiving blood from the artery of the womb (the twins shared a placenta). He was born very red because he had received more than his fair share of red blood cells and the other was pale and anaemic. But, although both children developed regressive autism-type symptoms, the pale one came good faster. Why? It was because the mother had multiple mercury containing amalgams when she carried the twins, and this mercury is known to 'leak' into the foetus, carried there by haemoglobin in the red blood cells.

To the mothers joy and amazement, this twin boy turned the corner rapidly when the alkalizing program began. Here was a sure and certain indicator to me that the new alkalizing technique had profound possibilities. I knew, from the Fenton science – taught me by heavy metal scientist Hans Rex, that mercury and other heavy metals would leave the body ('chelate') in an alkaline internal environment. Here was the evidence. A remarkable change after three years of otherwise only mild success.

Such a result showed us that alkalising alone can improve ASD — exciting!

However, even before this episode, my first indicators of the possibilities of this technique had been seen in an 8 year old ODD (oppositional defiant) girl of one family, and a 4 years old badly delayed (GDD) boy in another family who began to follow this program at the same time.

Both had what is called a 'healing crisis'; they both became worse, with return of their previous symptoms of bad and defiant behavior and opposition. Yet, after a period of feeling unwell and nausea, they turned the corner and 'came out the other side' with a very marked advancement in their ASD. Since this, we have seen many children and adults do the same (but we have learned to control the process so 'healing crisis' are now very rare).

Since then we have developed what appears to be a sound, easy-to-apply and low-cost pH program.

So, how do we elevate the pH and chelate effectively?

Instructions

We use a powder called 'Tri-Salts' (made up by a compounding chemist using 2506 mg sodium bicarbonate, 1651 mg potassium bicarb and 843 mg calcium carbonate, flavored with genuine apricot or mango!

and sweetened with Stevia) The kids like it. (Well, there will be a boy or girl who doesn't, I guarantee!).

You can also, very simple, buy sodium bicarbonate and citric acid from the supermarket or local store.

- Just mix 1.2 parts of sodium bicarb to one part citric acid. So, a teaspoon slightly rounded to a level teaspoon (citric acid actually has an alkalising effect in the body fluids).
- Use one teaspoonful of this mix in ½ litre of pure water (not tap water). Sweeten further with 'Stevia' – if necessary. Twice daily or as needed to maintain 7 pH (see below). One half-hour before meals or less – it does to appear to harm the digestive juices, but is best taken a little while before eating.
- Shake the bottle of powder well before mixing the dose into water.
- Take urine samples twice daily. Measure the pH with urine strips or a pH meter (see below). Aim for maintaining a 7+ reading. Adjust pH water intake as needed to keep that level.
- **Monitor your child for unusual symptoms**. Cut-back the alkalizing if nausea or unwellness or there is a sudden loss of ground (gained by therapy) to this date, for no other apparent reason.

pH meters or strips available

I use an electronic meter, which is very fast, accurate and has a virtual one-off price. You can buy them for around $90 (US). We can supply these from Australia, if necessary.

Strips that are accurate in a narrow pH range are hard to find, but I sourced some that will cost under 0.16 c cents per reading. 200 tests for $27 (US).

Another timing of this method is recommended by Dennis L. Myers, M.D. of Indiana, Pennsylvania:

> "The important thing is to take the (TriSalts or bicarb of soda and citric acid) on an empty stomach, so it can suck out the excess "deposit acid" from the acid producing cells lining the stomach (thereby generating more bicarbonate which goes into the blood stream) and not interfere with the acid that is needed at the times of eating. One needs acid in the stomach to digest food obviously so the Balanced Base Powder or baking soda should not be taken around meal times.
>
> If you eat breakfast at 8:00 A.M. and lunch at noon then you would take the first dose of Base Powder at 10:00 A.M., the same

between lunch and dinner. It is best to sip it even, so it can suck out acid from the stomach over a longer time, not all at once as with one big gulp. If there isn't time to sip it, just drink it anyway. This, done consistently, over time, is what makes the difference.

It is best not to eat before you retire at night. If you don't eat before bed time then you can take ½ to 1 tsp. of Base Powder before bed also. If you do eat before bed then you would not take the Base Powder that night.

To determine the amount of Base Powder you should take you should check your urine pH at the same times as you would take the Base Powder (don't take the Base Powder and check your urine on the same day), i.e. between meals, say at 10:00 A.M. or 2:00 P.M. The urine should be kept at a pH of 7.0 to 8.0 at all such times. If it is below this number, i.e. if it still acid then you need more Base Powder. If the pH stays between 7.0 and 8.0 then you can try to decrease the amount of powder."

Diet

An alkaline diet is the best way of helping maintain a good pH. Select from the – foods on the list. As you can see from the food list our modern diet is a pH disaster. My next book will contain a great deal more on this important pH subject.

The more negative the foods alkaline ranking, the more beneficial is the effect on these measures.

Acid Foods (+)

Grains: brown rice +12.5, rolled oats +10.7, whole wheat bread +8.2, spaghetti +7.3, corn flakes +6.0, white rice +4.6.

Dairy: parmesan cheese +34.2, processed cheese +28.7, hard cheese +19.2, cottage cheese +8.7, whole milk +0.7.

Legumes: peanuts +8.3.

Meats, Fish, Eggs: trout +10.8, turkey +9.9, chicken +8.7, eggs +8.1, beef +7.8.

Alkaline Foods (–)

Fruits: raisins –21.0, black currants –6.5, bananas –5.5, apricots –4.8.

Vegetables: spinach –14.0, celery –5.2, carrots –4.9, lettuce –2.5.

References

Frassetto, L.A., et al. 1996. Effect of age on blood acid-base composition in adult humans: Role of age-related renal function decline. American Journal of Physiology 271 (6-2): F1114-1122.

Sebastian, A., et al. 1994. Improved mineral balance and skeletal metabolism in postmenopausal women treated with potassium bicarbonate. New England Journal of Medicine 330 (25): 1776-1781.

Frassetto, L.A., et al. 1997. Potassium bicarbonate reduces urinary nitrogen excretion in postmenopausal women. Journal of Endocrinology and Metabolism 82 (1): 254-259.

Remer, T., and F. Manz. 1995. Potential renal acid load of foods and its influence on urine pH. Journal of the American Dietetic Association 95 (7): 791-797.

Joe Friel is the author of The Cyclist's Training Bible, The Triathlete's Training Bible, and Cycling Past 50. He is a certified coach by USA Cycling and USA Triathlon and has been coaching endurance athletes for two decades. He may be reached by email at jfriel@ultrafit.com.

CHAPTER EIGHT

Chelation in Alphabet Kids

Getting rid of heavy metals

Having now learned how to alkalise your child or yourself, we must now learn the new and simple ways to actually remove the heavy metals from the body – which process is called chelation.

Because of the following reasons, Chelation has often been a major problem for many, and in some aspects virtually impossible – especially for young autistic, oppositional defiant or hyperactive children:

- Expense
- Intravenuous (vein drips, for several hours) over multiple days
- Oral route – too large tablets/capsules for younger children
- Making of weeks of appointments
- Not always without side effects

Newly discovered chelation methods – rid your child of heavy metals

Simple, effective, low cost and safe – when supervised by a suitable practitioner

The origination of the word *chelation* helps understand its meaning! Coming from a Greek word for *clawing*, chelation literally means *to claw out* heavy metals.

Until very recently this has been a highly skilful medical process using special and expensive chemicals intravenously. These bio-chemically 'get hold' of metals like lead and mercury, and take them out of the body.

Using hair as a marker, and sending the sample to a specialist laboratory, we can tell if a child has heavy metals. Some metals, like aluminum are not accurate using this method – but the other major 'heavies' are reliably reported by a good laboratory (we use Doctors Data in Chicago or Great Smokies in North Carolina).

Over 2000 university and other clinical studies on chleation were available as long ago as 1984. Today they are voluminous. The interesting results of those studies showed patients with cardiovascular disease no longer needed bypasses and other expensive surgical operations. Yet modern hierarchical medicine only acknowledges its use for the heavy metal lead.

This success with cardio-vascular disease was bad news for heart surgeons.

Inevitably the "expert" spin-doctors began their strident chants in medical journals. Hand-in-hand with gullible worshipping journalists they danced with fancy-footwork around the cauldron of falsehood, pronouncing Chelation as "useless" or worse. I know, because I was involved in the first Chelation clinic in Australia in 1983 and saw the demise of a first-class clinic where many people's lives had been saved. (The 40 year old New Zealander whose vision started this clinic, had suffered a one sided paralysis stroke. He had Chelation in California, and regained full normality. I met him after his recovery). One of my doctor friends did a medical paper search on Chelation at the local hospital library. He found scores of anti-chelation material and not one of the medical studies that proved otherwise. Since that eye-opening time we have been informed of similar dishonest practices in many branches of medicine, including cancer, arthritis, diabetes and not the least – psychiatry, where their lies have now met the Courts in connection with suicide and homicide causing drugs. And their standard handbook on psychiatric symptoms (the so-called DMS series) has been called into question as doing more harm than good in some categories.

By 1986 we began to use a newly available oral version of Chelation. I remember my first patient, due for a by-pass in a few months, began the tablets and on his follow-up pre-op appointment with his cardiologist, was found problem-free. He was a bee-keeper from country Victoria.

Since then we have used oral Chelation, but also believed that the intravenous route was probably the best. So, we often sent people to the doctors who specialized in i.v. Chelation. Now we have new oral methods, and even cream-on-the-skin methods, that work <u>better</u> than the intravenous route!

For a very recent illustration of this success, one of our friends – also a client, with a long history of extremely painful vascular problems affecting both heart and head, began a series of intravenous chelation – using the conventional methods. He improved considerably, but it was a costly and long draw-out episode.

A few months after the series completed he found himself returning to symptoms again. This time he decided to try an oral route chelation. This worked to well, he told us that his symptoms began to improve within 24 hours of the first dose. He has been on this now for several months and is looking and feeling extremely well. It has cost him one third of the intravenous, with better results.

Soon we expect flak. This time from the doctors using i.v. Chelation!

Serendipity soup and Doctor Yoshiaki Omura

The best has been reserved until last, it seems. We now have the cheapest and most effective chelating agent ever found. Parsely! well — Chinese Parsely, best known to the western world as cilantro or coriander. The following is an account of its recent discovery by the very observant Dr Yoshiaki Omura:

> "Dr. Omura recently informed us that he discovered almost by accident, that the leaves of the coriander plant can accelerate the excretion of mercury, lead and aluminum from the body. He had been treating several patients for an eye infection called trachoma (granular conjunctivitis), which is caused by the micro-organism Chlamydia trachomatis. Following the standard treatment with antibiotics. Dr. Omura found that the patients' symptoms would clear up initially, then recur within a few months. He experienced similar difficulties in treating viral related problems like Herpes Simplex types I & II and Cytomegalovirus infection.
>
> After taking a closer look, Dr. Omura found those organisms seemed to hide and flourish in area of the body where there were concentrations of heavy metals like mercury, lead and aluminum. Somehow the organisms were able to use the toxic metals to protect themselves from the antibiotics."
>
> ### *Vietnamese Soup Flushed Out Heavy Metals!*
>
> It just so happens that while he was testing for those metals, Dr. Omura noticed the mercury level in the urine increased after one consumed a healthy serving of Vietnamese soup. The soup contains Chinese parsley, or it is better known in this country, cilantro. (Some of you may also know it as coriander, since it comes from the leaves of the coriander plant.)
>
> "Further testing revealed that eating cilantro also increased urinary excretion of lead and aluminum. And when cilantro was used concurrently with antibiotics or natural anti-viral agents and/ or fatty acids like EPA with D.A., the above infection could be eliminated for good. **(Acupnct Electrother Res. 95:20 (3-4): 195-229.)**

Dr Omura found that fresh cilantro removes heavy metals from the body in less than two weeks.

... but wait, there's more!

He also discovered that his patients had fewer colds and flu after removing the heavy metals because it seems that viruses and bacteria like to congregate in organs contaminated by heavy metals. In other words, the vital immune function of his patients was being optimized.

This chelating agent, along with a comprehensive program, is now being used by prestigious clinics (where Truth is allowed to grow, no matter were it comes from). One of these is part of the detox program of Dr Dietrich Klinghardt MD PhD of the American Academy of Neural Therapy, Institute of Neural Biotherapy, Washington State.

Now used by dentists in Australia for mercury reduction

A clinical scientist I know in the field of dentistry also uses and recommends the protocol of Dr Klinghardt. He is Dr David Gammal, of Sydney, founder of the Australian Oral Medicine & Toxicology Association. Dr Gammal is a well-known, much respected and well-liked pioneer in Australia of anti-mercury science and holistic dentistry.

The Institute of Neural Therapy in USA found that coriander is capable of mobilizing mercury, cadmium, lead, and aluminium in both the bones and the central nervous system. They found it is probably the only effective agent, to date, that will mobilize mercury stored in the intracellular space (space inside the cells), where mercury can attach to vital cell components.

To understand the essential need for chelation in many ASD children and adults, we need to realise that heavy metals like mercury, lead, arsenic, antimony and cadmium are real toxins that can affect a child's mind, nervous system and immune system – severely. Mercury (Hg) is the third most potent **neurotoxin** subtance known to man.

Neurotoxins **are poisons that are attracted to our nervous system because it contains substances like fatty acids (FA) which they like. These FA's make-up the bulk of the insulation that surrounds our nerve fibres.**

Heavy metals are all primarily neurotoxins. **There is an interacting (synergistic) effect between all neurotoxins which is responsible for worsening the illness producing effect. For instance, according to Professor Boyd Haley, head of chemistry at the University of Kentucky, and a leading expert on mercury, aluminum can potentate (make worse) the toxicity of mercury by several times.**

Unfortunately, aluminum (aluminum) is also found in many things we use (utensils) or put onto our bodies (anti-perspirants), and in vaccines.

No wonder then, that by making neurotoxin elimination a major part of our practice has led to some amazing results. Many other chronic illnesses besides autism spectrum disorders (e.g. Chronic fatigue, fibromyalgia, lupus) once considered intractable can respond when such related loads on the immune system are removed.

Dietrich Klinghardt, M.D., Ph.D. of the Neurobiology Institute says that:

> "**Neurotoxins** are absorbed by nerve endings and then travel inside the neuron to the cell body. On their way they disrupt vital functions of the nerve cell, such as axonal transport of nutrients, mitochondrial respiration and proper DNA transcription. **The body is constantly trying to eliminate neurotoxins** via the available exit routes: the liver, kidney, skin and exhaled air."

There are many natural detox mechanisms, but these can be overcome by large heavy metal loads that deplete the natural sacrificial chemicals and excreting pathways and by an acid cellular (internal)environment.

Detox for the liver

The liver is one of these detox mechanisms and will respond as it should when helped by a good liver enhancing herb or homeopathic treatment, as set out below.

In fact, the liver is the most important of all these mechanisms. Here most elimination products, including 90% of chelated mercury, are expelled with the bile into the small intestine and, with correct treatment, should leave the body via the digestive tract and large bowel. But without the total proper treatment (also described below), which you can do at home, some of the heavy metals can be reabsorbed by the abundant nerve endings of the intestinal nervous system in the gut walls. This is because there are more neurons here than in the whole spinal chord! And heavy metals are attracted to neurons.

This re-absorption can be avoided by simply taking a good spirulina or chlorella at the same time as the following oral chelation treatment. We use *Hawaiian Pacifica* **Certified Organic Spirulina.** This enhances the Chelation effect, stops most of the re-toxification, and shortens the time-span of treatment. We also use charcoal powder or tablets if there are signs of re-toxication (headaches, increase of autism spectrum symptoms, nausea, faintness, paleness, nervousness, weakness). Do not be concerned if these appear. Immediately give charcoal powder or tablets in or with milk plus more Spirulina powder or tablets. There should normally be no increase in temperature or pulse if this event happens at all.

Cease the Chelation program for two days and recommence at a lower rate of use

By following the amounts and directions below, you should have no problems.

The following home usage of oral chelation should be supervised by a suitable practitioner ...

No 1 It is essential drink plenty of water or drinks with water in them, as freshly made vegetable juices, homemade lemonade (no sugar – use 'Stevia' from health food store).
'Plenty' of water means 5 glasses of above daily for children, 10 glasses for adults.
This is essential for your bloodstream to 'flush' your body of wastes.
Do not allow "soft dinks'.

No 2 Morning meal must have protein in it (i.e. eggs; fish; soya beans or other legumes like chick peas; vegetarian sausages etc (see below). Proteins provide the raw material for your child's natural chelating agents.

No 3 Every meal should have minerals added. We use colloidal trace minerals and Celtic Salt or Dr Vogels vegetable salt or similar. These are also natural chelators.

No 4 Daily take twice the recommended use of broad-spectrum essential fatty acids (EFA's).

No 5 Go on the sugar-free program, using 'Stevia' in place of sugar. Do not use Aspartame.

No 6 **See your chemist for a short anti-fungal course of medicine.** Or, if in Australia, take 'Prograstrim' brand of bacteria.

No 7 Buy a herbal or homeopathic liver support or liver detoxicant. They are readily available. One often used is St Mary's Thistle (sylimarin).

The important natural chelating supplements

Spirulina or chlorella: A half-hour before meals (important) take 2–6 tablets (depending on size of child – you cannot over-do this, but small children don't like tablets), or one level teaspoon powder (in flavored juice, like apricot). IMPORTANT: This stops re-absorption of metals in small intestine. Otherwise, your child can develop some side-effects (not permanent – but the transient increase of his/her problems caused by heavy metals). (We recommend *Hawaiian Pacifica Certified* Spirulina and *Sun* Brand Chlorella)

Cilantro drops: Almost tasteless & quite pleasant. Commence with Two drops twice daily, take just before eating (IMPORTANT: ***a half-hour after the chlorella or Spirulina***). Gradually increase dose to 10 drops 3 times daily.

During the first six weeks of the detox, give one week 'on' and two weeks 'off'.

Other ways of using cilantro (coriander) is in cooking, below is a recipe for a Pesto:

Cilantro Pesto
1 clove garlic
1/2 cup almonds, cashews, or other nuts
1 cup packed fresh cilantro leaves
2 tablespoons lemon juice + 6 tablespoons olive oil
Celtic Sea Salt to taste (from health food store)
You can search for other ways.

Other efficient methods for children who don't like coriander or your nice Pesto

Trans-dermal method: You can also rub 3 drops into each wrist and into the ankles. This mobilizes the heavy metals in the upper and lower half of the body via the dense nerve networks and lymph channels, which can both absorb cilantro.

Drinking tea: Add 10 drops in a cup of hot peppermint tea, sweeten with Stevia, and sip this slowly, three times daily.

Selenium drops: 200 – 400 mcg daily. ***Two hours away from taking vitamin C.***

Vitamin C: 3–5 gms daily (3,000–6,000 mgm). Rule-of-thumb: 1000 mgm for every year of life until six years of age. Or, until 'bowel tolerance' – if he gets the 'runs', go back to a lesser amount. There will be no damage done. This amount of vitamin C has been given for many decades. Do not believe the propaganda from sources that cannot patent Vitamin C. Vitamin C actually protects the kidneys from kidney stones and has been found to dissolve bladder stones in dogs.

Colloidal minerals: two teaspoons daily

Magnesium and other electrolytes: add daily the recommended amount.

CHAPTER NINE

Finding the evidence

This section is for the scientifically minded!

In a previous Chapter I mentioned the little girl who refused a handful of sugar-rich jellybeans. Her doctor had said to the mother that *Candida* could not cause ADHD. It was that remark that led to this Chapter of investigation.

One exceptionally helpful contact has been Bernhard Hube Ph.D., from Hamburg University Dept. of Microbiology and a mycologist at the famous Robert Koch Infectious Diseases Institute in Berlin (Koch was the world-renowned Nobel Laureate bacteriologist of the late 19th century). Dr Hube is well-known for his molecular biology in the study of the virulence of candida. 'Virulence' in this case, means the ability of the organism to propagate, inhabit, invade tissue and migrate systemically (throughout the body). We established a correspondence. He showed some interest in my clinical findings and my requests for more precise information on what toxins were being released by the *Candida albicans* buds, especially as they became systemic. However, his work has 'only' been unravelling the ways in which candida ***commonly*** invades the body systemically (which commonality in the general population has been largely denied by orthodox medicine).

Other sources provided me with information on the mind/body toxins actually released once the invasion has taken place. These can be likened, in some cases, to the defecation we normally do in the toilet taking place in our bloodstream by candida buds. Or, in other cases, on death of the buds – of their corpses rotting and releasing their toxins. These toxins had been proved to cause extensive tissue damage by a study performed at Youngstown University in Ohio, 1994 (*Cytobios*, 1994, 77, 310:147-158) followed by an Australian study at the Division of Cell Biology, John Curtin School, Canberra (Waring & Beaver,*Gen Pharmacology*, 1996) which indicated gliotoxin to be 'a potent cause of cell death'.

Some of the known toxins associated with *C. albicans*

Among others, *Candida albicans* (c.a.) toxins include:

Agent	*Activity*
Canditoxin (exotoxin)	inflammatory; nerve-growth stimulator;
Mannan (cell wall layer)	immunosuppressive inhibits lymphocyte response to c.a.;
Zymosan (cell wall layer)	inflammatory, associated with psoriasis;
Ethanol (catabolic product)	alcoholic symptoms; produces acetaldehyde;
Acetaldehyde* (catabolic product)	tissue damage; abnormal behaviour/emotions;
Microbial Metabolites** (catabolic product)	Found to affect autism and ADHD
Unidentified systemic toxins	Wide range of symptoms linked to *Candida albicans*
Gliotoxin metabolite	Enzyme inhibitor; immunosuppresive; anti-phagocytic, anti-macrophagic; fragments DNA; many other toxic effects recorded ('Potent inducer of cell death', Division of Cell Biology, John Curtin School, Canberra, Australia)

* Acetaldehyde is formed by oxidation of ethanol, an alcohol produced by *C. albicans* when richly fed sugars. One American driver was arrested for being over-the-limit, despite being 'dry'. He was found to have heavy *candidiasis* that 'brewed' a high alcohol level. This was proved to the satisfaction of the court, and the case was dismissed. Acetaldehyde can cause the symptoms of most of the behavourial, emotional and learning difficulties found in children. The aldehyde group Arabinose can cross-link with the amino acid arginine, to alter the biological structure and function of many proteins (*J. Biological Chemistry*, 264:21597-21602, 1989). This means it is possible that biological changes can occur, affecting tissue functions.

** Microbial metabolites: in a 1100 patient retrospective analysis presented to the First International Conference on Chronic Fatigue Syndrome in 1989 (Jessup MD), it was shown that these patients had been treated for nine years for chronic fatigue, dizziness, depression, headache, night sweats, arthralgias, myalgias (muscle soreness after working) and stiffness in the morning.

About 80% of these people had repeated antibiotic treatment for acne, respiratory or urinary tract infections; 60% had developed sensitivity to antibiotics. Alcohol intolerance, irritable bowel syndrome, recurrent vaginitis, migraine headaches, skin disease and PMT were frequent complaints. Almost all had sugar or alcohol craving prior to the onset of chronic fatigue. Treatment had shown little improvement and 685 were unemployed due to *candidiasis* infection, and receiving disability pensions. Dr Jessup began treating them with an anti-candida medicine combined with a regime free of alcohol, sugars, fruit or juice.

How *C. albicans* invades our body and bloodstream

This is what the researchers have found:

> Until recently it was thought throughout the community studying and/or treating candida problems, that the yeast buds could not invade mucosal linings until they developed into the mycelial thread-like or hypha (web) form. This mycelial form was thought to be the most virulent. But this understanding has been described as simplistic by Frank Odds, the respected director of mycology (science of fungi) at the Janssen Research Foundation in Belgium. The common dogma, as he put it, is that the hyphae put out feelers that burrowed into the tissue by "spewing out broad-spectrum hydrolytic (dissolving) enzymes along their track to overcome the hosts array of antimicrobial factors". (*Candida Species and Virulence,* 1994)

In his paper published in the *Journal of Mycology* (1998), Dr Bernard Hube presents a more up-to-date understanding of the tricky ways in which candida albicans actually operates.

He points out that the last eight years of research around the world have located at least nine members of an enzyme-family called aspartyl proteinases. These are secreted by the yeast buds and are labelled 'secreted aspartyl proteinases' (produced by genes SAP 1–9). These are Smart Guys. The Top Gun is SAP 2, which produces the family members that have the most ability to degrade proteins like collagen and mucin, thus making it possible to invade our gut. SAP 2's can also invade endothelial cell layers – cells that line the blood vessels, heart and other body cavities. A more recent study (Martin Schaller, et al) has found SAP1-3 causing tissue necrosis (destruction) in epithelial tissue. Epithelial tissue is the outer wall of our vascular system.

Even a simple yeast bud can penetrate our tissues

This means that the 'simple' yeast form buds can invade our bloodstream via the outer and inner vascular walls without having to 'switch' into hyphae format, although hyphae/mycelial thread forms also produce SAP's. Once systemic they can produce the potent toxins described above and produce many of the symptoms so common in candidiasis. Among them ADHD and ADD.

Not only can the SAP's invade certain places where their host-bud (or hyphae form) may land, but if the niche happens to be a comparatively high pH (a hostile environment for yeast forms) they can produce members of their family called SAP's 4 –6 which are active at near neutral pH (like your mouth). The Smart Guys from the SAP 2 side of the family can also degrade the immune system by destroying immunoglobulins like IgA and macroglobulins.

The research has confirmed that *C. albicans* can do all can kinds of fancy footwork, side-stepping, accelerating, switching and changing direction like a highly paid football striker running in for a Grand Final winning score. Like the footballer, the best way to stop *candida* is to starve him of what keeps him moving! In this case sugars and other simple carbohydrates (e.g. typically white bread).

All this work has been even more recently confirmed by a paper published in *Molecular Microbiology* in August, 1999. This showed beyond doubt that *C. albicans* buds themselves invade human tissue by means of the Smart Guy SAP's without help from hyphae forms. Once there, they proceed to produce their SAP virulence for further damage, as shown by antigen-antibody studies in 1997 (B. Hube et al. *Infect Immun*, 65:3259-3538).

Any doctor who tells you that yeast buds cannot invade into the blood-stream (become systemic) and cause multiple symptoms, is not up-to-date.

Antibiotics and acute middle-ear infection (AOM)

To re-cap our journey: we have found that a common route takes these children to the symptoms in the Questionnaire (see page 251). Beginning with milk sensitivus, respiratory/skin infections and middle-ear infection. Traditionally these patients have been treated with anti-biotics, despite the fact that children have the fastest growing resistance to anti-biotics of any group in our population.

In a study of 518 children with ear infection, Cantekin (*J. American Medical Assocation,* 266, 1991) found that six weeks after stopping the antibiotic amoxicillin, recurrence was 2-6 times higher in the antibiotic-treated children than those in the placebo group. Van Buchem treated one group of otitis media patients with antibiotics, one with tubes in the ears, and a third with neither. The outcome in the three groups was essentially the same (Van Buchem, F. and Dunk, J. *Therapy of acute otitis media: myringotomy, antibiotics, or neither?* Lancet 2: 883-887, 1981).

As we have found, the anti-biotics cause internal problems by upsetting the gastro-intestinal balance between friendly bacteria (that are significantly reduced by anti-biotics) and yeast-forms that do not respond to anti-biotics. This significantly affects the immune system. Typically, recurring respiratory and middle-ear (otitis media – OM) infections commence. Repeated OM infections have been linked to ADD-HD in many studies. Here are three sample studies:

Otitis Media in children with learning disabilities and in children with ADHD

Based on parental report, children with ADD-H had significantly more complaints of earaches during the preceding 3 months and significantly more ear infections during the preceding year.

Although middle ear disease in preschool children has repeatedly been linked to later language deficits, this study suggests that middle ear disease in school-age children may also be associated with hyperactivity and/or inattention, independently of learning disability.

Adesman AR, Altshuler LA, Lipkin PH, Walco GA.
Pediatrics, 1990 Mar, 85(3 Pt 2):442-6.
Division of Developmental and Behavioural Pediatrics,
Schneider Children's Hospital, Long Island Jewish Medical Center, New Hyde Park, NY 11042

Minimal brain dysfunction and Otitis Media

The frequency of otitis media among 22 hyperactive children with learning disorders was compared with the frequency of otitis media in a sample of 772 normal children, using the same criteria for the diagnosis of otitis media in both groups. The groups were matched for social class and age (7–13 years of age). A significantly higher percentage of hyperactive children (54%) had more than 6 episodes of otitis media than was found in the normal group (15%). Thirty-six percent of hyperactive children had more than 10 episodes compared to 5% in the normal sample.

Hersher L., Percept Mot Skills, 1978 Dec; 47(3 Pt 1):723-6

An association between recurrent Otitis Media in infancy and later hyperactivity

Subjects were 67 children referred to a child development clinic for evaluation of school failure. Ranging from 6 to 13 years old, all the children demonstrated specific school learning problems, and 27 were also considered hyperactive by two or more raters. Sixteen of the hyperactive children were treated with central nervous system stimulant medication.

In retrospect, there was a positive correlation between an increasing number of otitis media infections in early childhood and the presence and severity of hyperactive behaviour. Ninety-four percent of children medicated for hyperactivity had three or more otitis infections, and 69 percent had greater than 10 infections. In comparison, 50 percent of non-hyperactive school-failure patients had three or more infections and 20 percent had greater than 10 infections. Twenty-two of 28 children (79%) known to have more than 10 infections experienced recurrent otitis before 1 year of age

Hagerman RJ, Falkenstein AR. Pediatr (Phila) 1987 May; 26(5):253-7

The direct connection of infections, candida & ADD/H

Although all three studies recognised an association between OM infections and ADHD, none of them gave any hint as to what might be the mechanism that caused ADHD to develop.

In my considered opinion, based on the rapid disappearance of ADHD symptoms in the now thousands of children many paediatricians and practitioners like myself have treated among us to date, it is becoming plain that the common denominator is not the infections but the ***results of treating those infections with antibiotics***, namely candidiasis, another infection. The mechanism for this is well-known and, with advancing discoveries in molecular biology and biochemical pathology, fits the picture accurately. This view has been confirmed positively since writing this section, by the prestigious Great Plains Laboratory in USA, whose chief biochemistry pathologist Dr William Shaw has stated:

> "Kontstantareas and Homatidis at the University of Guelph in Ontario, Canada found a high correlation between the prevalence of ear infections and the incidence of autism. They found that the earlier the child had an ear infection, the more likely that child had of a more severe form of autism. Many similar studies have

been conducted in the field of attention deficit hyperactivity (ADHD). These studies also indicate that increased ear infection early on in life results in much greater incidents of hyperactivity.

Roberts and his colleagues reported that recurrent otitis media (OM) during infancy was correlated with increased distractibility of the students later in life. Other studies correlated recurrent OM in infancy with later low IQ scores, poor performance on tests of reading, spelling, and math, increased retention in grade, increased attention deficits, and increased behaviour problems in school.

Both the autism and ADHD research groups have assumed that the hearing impairment caused by the ear infection is what caused the abnormal development. My own interpretation of these data is that abnormal by-products of yeast and drug-resistant bacteria absorbed into the body from the intestine following the excessive use of antibiotics is the cause of these epidemics."

It is interesting to note that ADHD children who respond to the treatment described in this book, which in my group has been 90%, do not have residual hearing problems and their learning/behaviour improves significantly. This indicates that there was no *abnormal development* in the first place – only *abnormal internal function.*

CHAPTER TEN

More on the Leaky Gut

When your child's internal filter is damaged

As with your tongue, the healthy intestine is lined on the surface with 'wet' mucosal cells that form the surface of the tiny 'fingers' called micro-villi through which digested food components are transported or diffused into the bloodstream. This mucosa is protected by a huge population of specialist friendly bacteria (probiotics). In fact, a healthy adult should have around 1½ kilos of these various probiotics. At about 10 billion per gram that equals 1500 x 10 billion bacteria, and without them we would not survive. (Humbling, isn't it!) Antibiotics seriously reduce this vital population and allow *candida* species and other pathogens to colonize.

When *Candida albicans* proliferates it produces the secreted enzymes (described in the previous Chapter) that can 'eat' their way through this mucosal and deeper collagen base tissue, so enlarging normal filtered absorption areas to allow larger than usual food particles into the blood-stream. This complicates the *candida* invasion further, as now the food particles are seen as 'enemies' by specialist immune cells and begin a reaction against them. This is a food allergy or sensitivity. We now have both *C. albicans* toxins plus allergens invading the blood-stream. As a result our patients invariably have numerous food sensitivities, although not always aware of them – they cause some of the chronic tiredness always found. Until we can repair the intestinal wall and control the *C. albicans* we find it useless to even identify these allergies (although obvious major problem foods must be removed – but these are usually already identified by the astute mothers).

Other parasitic and bacterial organisms, like antibiotic resistant *streptococcus, cryptosporidium* and *campylobacter* are sometimes involved but do not appear to behave in the same way as yeast in producing ADD/H symptoms.

Your child's best (micro-)friends!

The infant and childhood gut is normally protected from these pathogenic bacteria/fungal/yeast forms by specialised friendly *lactobacillus* species only found in babies, infants and children to about 7 years of age. (Around seven to eight years the bacteria begin to change to adult type lactobacillus species). The infant bacteria arrive there via their journey through the mother's birth canal. Early studies showed that approximately 60% of four-to six-day old full-term babies born vaginally were colonized by *Bifidobacterium infantis* in contrast to only 9% born caesarean section (Natasha Trenev, *Probiotics, 1998)*.

Bifidobacterium infantis is the most important of the infant bacteria population. It should comprise 99% of the infant's bowel flora in the large intestine. Although, as mentioned before, *B. infantis* is very powerful in its ability to deal with dangerous organisms like *E. coli, Klebsiella* and *Salmonella* it is less robust than the other probiotics. It cannot cope so well with such problems as food chain pollutants, large scale *Candida* infections, air contaminants and anti-biotics.

The depletion of *B. infantis* is always accompanied by an increase in pathogenic bacteria and yeasts. Fortunately, this loss can be regained by use of powders that are made from live-strains of cultured *B. infantis* species given orally. In our Clinic we use the high quality Natren probiotics. The founder of Natren, Natasha Trenev was raised in former Yugoslavia, in a family with many generations of experience in the yoghurt industry. She later set-up a high tech research laboratory in California to study the intestinal flora believed to lie behind the longevity and good health of several nations in the Balkans and southern Russia. Today she is an acknowledged world expert in the growing and packaging of super-probiotic strains that can re-populate the human intestine. Probiotic research found that yoghurts often do not contain the specific human strains of *L. acidophilus, B. bifidum* and *L. bulgaricus*, we and our children need to re-populate the gut.

Speeding up the immigration process

Sometimes when necessary, we teach mothers who come to our clinic to use probiotics over the vulva area as well as rectally. To do this, we supply a 50mL catheter-tipped syringe fitted with a douche. This will nearly always speed-up the restoration process and is particularly effective in ending vaginal thrush in adults. These bacteria re-colonise and stimulate the immune system in a number of ways (*Micro-organisms used as probiotics*, Jeremija Rasic Ph.D., Faculty of Technology, Food Research Institute, Novi Sad, Yugoslavia). This is one of the most important methods we use to restore the damage done to the intestines by an anti-biotic assault. The method works for both adults and children, although the types of bacteria and their species differ.

Summary

Yeast forms multiply, invade the bloodstream and release toxins. These are often manifested in skin infections (see below). Later, migrating small lumps can appear, showing themselves on different places under the skin. Itching, or annoying and sometimes breaking into sores. (We often see this in the children attending our Clinic.) In one case, *Alopecia universalis* developed in a child who had been treated with repeated series of numerous anti-biotics. (*Universalis* is total body hair loss, which in this instance had lasted for two years).

Treating him for candidiasis brought improvement in his health and behaviour (he was also ADHD) in three days. In five months his hair had begun to grow again. But much of that was due to use of a German natural hair growth restorer (available from our clinic). This can even regrow hair from hair follicles that have been dormant for three or four years (as I proved on myself) as long as they are not irrevocably damaged.

More infections occur because milk products are still being used in the sensitive children and the anti-biotic induced yeast growth is causing sugar demand and compromising the immune system. (William Crook MD, *The yeast connection*, Jackson TN, Professional Books,1984)

Sugar depletes immune response. Phagocyte activity decreases with large or even moderate amounts of sugars.[63] Sugar can also cause skin problems and eczema in children.[64] By feeding the sugar-hungry candida and other sugar loving pathogens, sugar also causes fermentation in the bowel.[65]

Excess sugars upset the calcium-phosphorous balance, leading to 'bad nerves'. After many months of this internal warfare the virulent yeast forms begin to affect the brain and other organs.[66] They do this by releasing toxins, in particular acetaldehyde (a by-product of ethanol alcohol, itself a by-product of the candida's use of sugars). Acetaldehyde causes behavourial problems plus learning, comprehension and emotional problems; memory loss, distorted thinking, mood swings, depression, impaired intellectual functioning and abnormal behaviour (Dr William Crook MD, *Your guide to the world of alternative mental health* – Dr Crook is a respected and experienced paediatrician and author of the ground-breaking book *The Yeast Connection*).

According to the *Journal of Pediatrics Research* (38,4 (1995):539-542), sugar can also "worsen the symptoms of children with ADD". But I believe that it is the *C. albicans* that feeds on the sugars and produces the toxins that then worsen the symptoms of ADD. I say this because, once such a child has been on our anti-candida diet and treatment and has followed the gastro-intestinal improvement program for 3 months and taken our immune boosting Transfer Factor, sugar can be re-introduced carefully and there will be no worsening of ADD.

Moreover, Dr William Shaw during recently conducted important research on yeast and its effects on autism (ibid. *Your Guide* above) also found a marked decrease in hyperactive behaviour and better concentration when the *C. albicans* was treated.

These by-products of sugar breakdown via the *C. albicans* processing plant can also lead to vertigo (dizziness), sometimes severe. We have seen this on many occasions over the years, usually on waking. At different times during our live-in hospital days, we had three women who had reported early morning vertigo so severe they would fall over if rising from bed. Clearing their *C. albicans* problem cured the vertigo. The scientific literature has noted a connection with dizziness and sugar consumption.[67]

A note to mothers: adults can also, of course, be victims of candidiasis. Some of the mothers who bring their children relate to the Questionnaire themselves. Candida overgrowth can also be a common cause of chronic depression, especially in women between the ages of 25–45. This depression is caused by the toxic by-products of the candidiasis and other pathogens.

However, although highest on the list, candidiasis is only one of many possible causes. If you suspect *C. albicans*, remember that it is always accompanied by some or all of the several symptoms mentioned in this book, especially thrush – yet not always so. It is best to see a practitioner who understands *C. albicans*.

To test yourself for sugar craving, take this test

	True	False
I do not eat refined sugar every day.	☐	☐
I cant go for more than a day without eating some type of sugar-containing food.	☐	☐
I never have cravings for sugar, coffee, chocolate, peanut butter, or alcohol.	☐	☐
I've never hidden candy or other sweets around my home in order to find and eat them later.	☐	☐
I can stop after eating one piece of candy or one bite of pastry.	☐	☐

There are times when I have no sugar of any kind in my home.	☐	☐
I can go for three or more hours without eating and not experience the shakes, fatigue, perspiration, irritability, depression, or anxiety.	☐	☐
I can have candy and other sweets in my home and not eat them.	☐	☐
I do not eat something sweet after each meal.	☐	☐
I rarely drink coffee and eat donuts or sweet rolls for breakfast.	☐	☐
I can go for more than an hour after waking up in the morning without eating.	☐	☐
I can go from one day to the next without drinking a sweetened soft drink	☐	☐

Result

More than four 'False' replies = sugar cravings, with ascending significance after four

Studies that prove ADHD responds better to diet and candida control than to Ritalin

In October 1994, the monthly journal *Autism Research Review*, included a questionnaire response from 8,700 parents who had been trialing various drugs and other interventions to improve their children's problems (several of which are also common to ADHD and ADD children). The Report pointed out:

> "The 31 drugs listed first were prescribed by the child's physician in each case. Note that Ritalin, the drug most often prescribed, is near the bottom of the list. Only 26 % of the parents reported improvement, while 46% said the child got worse on Ritalin."

Examination of the study shows the anti-candida drug Nystatin ranked higher than any other prescription drug. Of the 208 children given one of the 31 drugs, 49% did better on the Nystatin and only 4% did worse. This is a better/worse ratio of more than 12:1. (Today we know that even Nystatin is not the best therapy for control of candidiasis. It is only temporary and can worsen the *Candida* problem if prolonged.)

Ritalin showed a better/worse ratio of 0.5:1. This means twice as many children were made worse by Ritalin than were helped! Moreover, the fact that treatment of candidiasis brought improvement in half of the children, underscores the toxicity problems produced by *C. albicans.*

Dr Crook described how he sent questionnaires to 16 doctors who were interested in the management of children with ADHD. Five found the anti-yeast therapy very effective, eight said it was somewhat effective, one said not effective and another did not try. So, 13 out of 15 doctors found a good to reasonable response in managing ADHD by using the anti-candida method. But Dr Crook goes on to say that later (in the 1950's) he found several foods that were common trouble-makers, causing similar symptoms, especially milk, wheat, corn, chocolate and egg. (See Appendix IX, 'Resources', for his excellent books on food allergy and candidiasis.)

CHAPTER ELEVEN

'Sugar blues' and other dangerous foods

This book has told you about the role sugar plays in the development and continuation of ASD problems and how in a long-term study of 3,486 ASD children 47% got better by removing sugars (see ARI chart at beginning of Part 2). We have shown how sugar can cause depression and also, paradoxically, hyperactivity. All refined sugars (glucose, table sugar, icing sugar, brown sugar, syrups etc) can become addictive. They are dangerous in large amounts. Way back in 1973, the Australian Minister for Health Dr John Everingham described sugar as 'a second rate food, a third rate drug and a third rate poison'. This, coming from a Government minister in one of the world's largest sugar producing countries, was a strong statement. He had good science behind him.

In 1943 endocrine physician and researcher Dr John Tintera discovered that patients suffering from hypoadrenocorticism (inadequate production of cortical hormones such as adrenaline) had the same symptoms as hypoglycaemic people, those with low-blood sugar. A common complaint today, those susceptible to low blood sugar problems are often fatigued, nervous, depressed, apprehensive, cant concentrate, or handle alcohol and have allergies, low blood pressure and a sugar craving. This was found when looking through the results of two hundred cases of the adrenal problem.

The conclusive test for this problem is called the glucose tolerance test (GTT). He ordered four hour GTT for all his patients on the trial. The results caused a stir in the pathology laboratory. They double-checked their results and then apologised for what they thought must be an error. This puzzlement came from the fact that the GTT was, until then, only used for adults with possible diabetes. Their tests for Dr Tintera had been done on adolescents with behavioural and mental problems. Dr Tintera wrote:

> 'These conditions might seem to arise or become aggravated at puberty (as in schizophrenia), but probing the patient's past will frequently reveal indications of these symptoms through pre-school and primary school years.
>
> A glucose tolerance test could alert parents and physicians and could save innumerable hours and small fortunes spent in looking in to the child's psyche and home environment."

He noted that 'obstinate resentment of discipline' (Opposition Defiant Disorder, or ODD as we call it today) and hyperactivity "are absolute indications for urinalysis (for sugars) and a 5-hour glucose tolerance test".

He also noted that drug addiction, alcoholism and schizophrenia were often found to be symptoms of the hyperadrenocorticism (producing too much adrenaline) individual.

Today we know that one of the chief characteristics of the alcoholic is Type A personality, the kind who have an almost obsessional drive in all they do, the 'adrenal flowing' person. If this personality does not feed correctly, is not fuelled-up with good all round nutrition then problems can occur. Too often, this type of person is a fast-fooder and sugar-freak. Unfortunately, serious problems can result.

Sugars and caffeine overdose – poison in a cup

I was involved in treating a typical case Type A hypoadrenocorticism several years ago. He was a young multi-millionaire, making his fortune in his own business enterprise. Daily he would faithfully keep himself fit by a long swim and a run on the beach. But his time for eating was limited to the minimum. One day after his usual swim and run he collapsed on the beach and had to be taken to hospital. He never really recovered. His adrenal system had failed. He became super-allergic, to the point where he could not be interviewed in a normal setting. It had to be outside in the fresh air, otherwise he was so distressed with allergies he found it hard to breath.

He lived on sugared coffee and diet-coke. I added his caffeine intake and found he was taking three times a medicinal dosage daily, and very little food – for several years. When he came to the doctors where I was working we found we could do little for him.

The whiter the bread, the sooner you're dead!

In 1978 I tested white bread and genuine wholemeal on guinea pigs. They were in the same box, with a partition between. The white-bread guinea pigs spent their life trying to get to their next door neighbours for a good feed. They eventually became ill and died.

Some bread manufacturers have a history of propaganda based on facts about as useless as some of the bleached flour they make. White flour is a poor food because it lacks most of the minerals, B vitamins and all of the essential vitamin E. For those children who can tolerate gluten breads, parents can check the chart below to gain some idea of the best bread to buy. These good breads are available in most supermarkets.

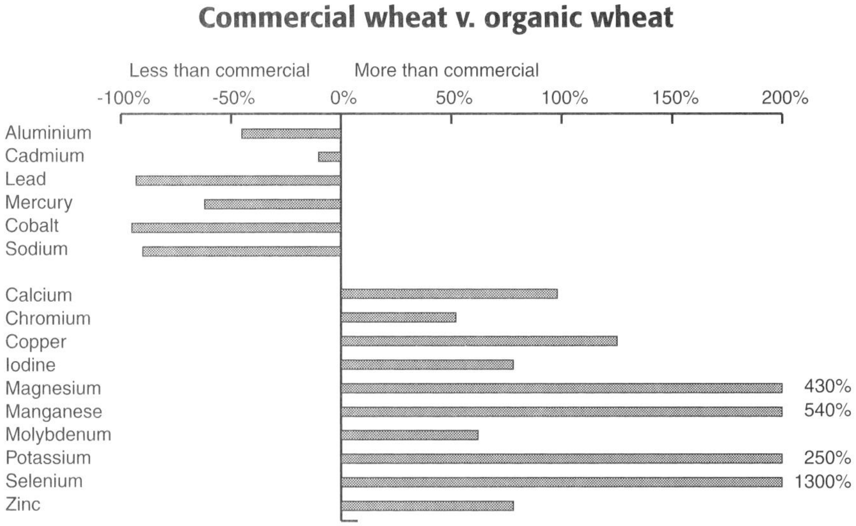

Adapted from The Journal of Applied Nutrition, 35;11993

Apparently, all food is not created equal. This study showed that organic wheat appears to have far more of the beneficial trace elements and less of the harmful trace metal contaminants.

Margarine – the doubtful & harmful spread

Do not use margarine!

In a well-known long-term study by Harvard University in 1994, 85,000 women were questioned about their dietary fat ingestion. The study found that those who used margarine had twice as much risk of heart disease as those who used butter. In another study of 1,250 women in 1999, researchers found a thirty per cent risk of breast cancer amongst women who ate margarine regularly compared with those who did not eat margarine. Even eating margarine a few times monthly increased the breast cancer risk by ten percent.

In another study, this time in New Zealand (Dr Patricia Holborow, University of Wellington, 1983) melanomas were found to be significantly linked to margarine consumption. The study was comparing all dietary intakes.

Moreover, melanomas have increased by more than fifty-fold since 1972, around the time that margarine began to be popularised. Coincidence? Maybe, maybe not. A study would have to discount many other factors as possible causes, before margarine could be directly linked to the rise.

These facts have been known for years, but few know them.

So, why is margarine so bad? Have you ever stopped to think how fluid oils become solid lumps? Why they are bright yellow? Taste unlike any oil? Don't go rancid? Look like butter? Stay soft? Spread so easy?

To make this metamorphosis happen the oils and other fats are first heated to around 150 °C in the presence of a metallic catalyst for some hours, which turns them black. It also changes the 'good fats' (cis fatty acids) into another chemical fat never before been seen by man, containing unhealthy trans fatty acids. Although this becomes a kind of monosaturated fat (usually considered a healthy fat), because of its unique chemical composition, it cannot be legally called such. It is more like a plastic polymer. And black! Now bleaching, flavouring, colouring and spreading agents are added. Margarine is not a natural product and, in the opinion of many experts, should be avoided. Use a good butter like Mainland instead.

Supermarket or mass produced chickens

If your family regularly eats chicken meat, it is strongly advised that you find a genuine free-range source. This especially applies to those with children who are endeavouring to improve their digestive and gut tracts. For more information, see the numerous consumer guides to healthy eating, or for a starting place see www.consumerreport.org, the US Consumers Union.

CHAPTER TWELVE

Genuine immunity versus vaccine immunity

"Disease is not mere surrender ... but also fight for health; unless there is fight there is no disease."

Medical pioneer Hans Selye M.D.
discoverer of 'stress syndrome'

The laws of nature can teach us lessons in how to raise a child with a strong immune system – help a chick break out of its egg, and you'll have an invalid chicken. It needs the struggle to get strong.

Grow agave (sisal) plants in well watered, rich soil – and you'll have no hard fibres for making rope. They need a tough fight, in poor soil and hot sun to make strong filaments.

Passively vaccinate a child and you'll have a child with a weak immune system. They need to fight with natural infections to develop strong immunity.

But a strong immune system is impossible if the necessary nutrients are not available. Vitamin C, the Prince of the Immune System – must be strongly there, along with several other key nutrients ...

Here is what the respected American medical and homeopathic doctor Richard Moskowitz MD wrote on the need for children to meet challenges their own way:

> "Childhood illnesses like measles, mumps and chicken pox produce symptoms which reflect the efforts of the immune system to clear the virus from the blood, which it does by sending it out exactly the same way it came in. When a child recovers from measles, you have true immunity. That child will never, never again get the measles no matter how many epidemics he is exposed to. Furthermore, he will respond vigorously and dramatically to whatever infectious agents he is exposed to. The side benefit of that disease is a non-specific immunity that charges or primes his immune system so that it can better respond to the subsequent challenges that it is going to meet in the future.
>
> Now, by contrast, when you take an artificially attenuated measles vaccine and introduce it directly into the blood and bypass the portal of entry, there is no period of sensitization of the

portal of entry tissues. There is no silent period of incubation in the lymph nodes. Furthermore, the virus itself has been artificially weakened in such a way that there is no generalized inflammatory response. By tricking the body in this way, we have done what the entire evolution of the immune system seems to be designed to prevent. We have placed the virus directly and immediately into the blood and given it free and immediate access to the major immune organs and tissues without any obvious way of getting rid of it.

The result of this, indeed, is the production of circulating antibodies, which can be measured in the blood. But that antibody response occurs purely as an isolated technical feat, without any generalized inflammatory response or any noticeable improvement in the general health of the organism. Quite the contrary, in fact. I believe that the price we pay for those antibodies is the persistence of virus elements in the blood for long periods of time, perhaps permanently, which in turn presupposes a systematic weakening of our ability to mount an effective response not only to measles but also to other infections. So far from producing a genuine immunity, the vaccine may act by interfering with or suppressing the immune response as a whole in much the same way as radiation and chemotherapy, corticosteroids and other anti-inflammatory drugs do.

Chronic long-term persistence of viruses and other proteins within cells of the immune system produce chronic disease. We know that live viruses are capable of surviving or remaining latent within host cells for years without continually provoking acute disease. They do this by attaching their own genetic material to the cell, and replicate along with the cell. That allows the host cell to continue its normal functioning but continuing to synthesize the viral protein.

Latent viruses produce various kinds of diseases. Because the virus is now permanently incorporated within the genetic material of the cell, the only appropriate immunological response is to make antibodies against the cell, no longer against the virus. So, immunizations promote certain types of chronic diseases. And far from providing a genuine immunity, the vaccines are actually a form of immunosuppression."[24] (Gratefully used, by permission.)

Although written nearly twenty years ago, this short thesis by a thinking doctor has proved all too true. In October 2001, another thoughtful and respected doctor – the paediatrician Philip Incao M.D., wrote this:

> "A growing number of scientists believe that the increase in America, Europe, Australia and Japan in allergic and auto-immune diseases (which stimulate the humoral or Th2 branch of the immune system) is caused by the lack of stimulation of the cellular (the Th1 branch) because of the lack of acute inflammatory responses and discharges in childhood. We need to identify the factors which cause this shift in the function of the immune system or which cause allergies and auto-immune diseases in childhood to increase!"[25]

Today, since the above was written, it has become obvious from both experience and the literature that immune system deficiency triggered by vaccination is a prime cause of acute middle-ear infection in many children. As an illustration, this week a client brought 12-year old Nathan in to see me. Nathan is third among four siblings. He began to regress soon after strong reactions to DTP vaccine. He is now ADHD and also has Aspergers symptoms.

Because of this, his mother did not allow vaccination for her last child (now 9 years of age). All the children except this last child had developed measles, whooping cough and multiple acute middle-ear infections, despite (or because of?) their vaccinations.

This family underscores what Dr Incao was saying: that children were 'missing' their normal important immunity challenges provided by a natural exposure to measles, mumps and whooping cough etc (and now, chicken pox). They were missing their fight with the natural exposure to the viruses.

But to win the necessary fight the immune system must be kept strong. It is like a 'camel with a load'. Too many straws and it collapses. The last straw can even break its back. However, removing straws early enough allows it to stand up. (With thanks to the memory of paediatrician Dr 'Billy' Crook who often used this illustration). Those early multiple deaths were caused by immune systems overloaded like the camel with crowded rooms for a whole family, stinking air from sewage, infected milk in open pails, questionable water supplies and poor nutrition.

The graph on the next page shows how an improved immune system can deal with even severe infectious childhood diseases. As you can see, the mortality rate among Australian infants was 130 per 1,000 live births in 1881. This fell to 57 per 1,000 live births between 1881 and 1932. This was a 43% drop in infant deaths due to these diseases in 50 years. This drop occurred before immunisation began and continued to fall at the same rate ***after*** vaccinations began. Since it was not immunisation that brought this dramatic change – what was it?

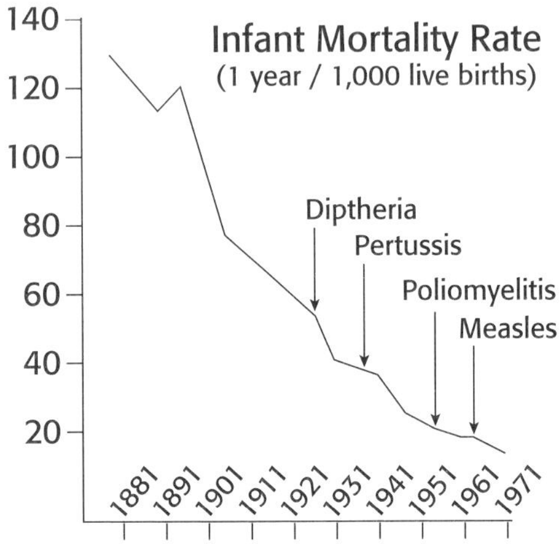

Courtesy of Maureen Hickman, "Vaccination – The Right Choice?" – sources: Australian Bureau of Statistics; NSW Public Health Bulletin, August-September, 1997

A clue to this lies in the fact that other Western nations achieved similar results in the same time frame. The common factor was the Government introduction of hygiene laws. Better housing, cleaner water, piped sewage, dairy hygiene and bottled milk (previously sold in open pails carried around the often filthy city streets). One Scottish medical director said that prior to this there was "diphtheria in every glass of milk" (Dr Leslie Mackenzie, member of the Scottish Medical Board, 1903). In Australia, bottled milk began in the late 1920's, and you can see this reflected in an even steeper downward curve in mortality at that time.

Advice for mothers who don't wish to vaccinate

In the normal course of events, when a child is exposed to a common infection like measles the virus enters through the doorways of the mouth or nose. In those sites the body has massive defences, and can quickly begin to mount an attack with a cellular response (white cells). This requires a preparation of nearly two weeks (the dormant stage). In this period the T helper cells are promoting a mobilization campaign, calling up the troops (as it were). Then, on the twelfth to fourteenth day the soldiers march into battle and the good fight begins. The child develops a gradually rising fever, loses his appetite and gets drowsy all day. Mucus discharge begins. Coughing begins. At that stage she is infectious to others for a week. (Some mothers purposely take their children to a neighbour who has measles occurring among their children). The temperature will rise even higher after the first two days and may reach over 41°C. Then the measles rash appears. To speed that good process, give your child a warm bath with a few tablespoons of Epsom salts dissolved in the water (even a half kilo is not too much). This "Brings Out" the rash, and can also be used for other rash-like diseases like chicken-pox. And even mumps. **This action can *really* increase the healing time, because you are helping your child's body in its task of repelling the invasion via the skin.**

This is a good thing happening

Let it be indelibly printed on your mind – this is all a good thing. The child's immune system is at work. After it's all over, the child will be stronger than before. As Dr Incao told the US Congress Sub-Committee in sworn statements:

> "I observed that my unvaccinated children were healthier, hardier and more robust than their vaccinated peers. Allergies, asthma and pallor and behavioural and attention disturbances were clearly more common in my young patients who were vaccinated. My unvaccinated patients, on the other hand, did *not* suffer from infectious diseases with any greater frequency or severity than their vaccinated peers: their immune systems generally handled these challenges very well."

Our own daughter was one who was never vaccinated. She had a severe measles fight, but has since then had excellent health. She had one brush with glandular fever at 16, but we requested a doctor friend to give her vitamin C intravenously. This procedure was carried out a day after pathology had identified the Epstein-Barr virus (that causes glandular fever). And given again the following day – Friday. The fever left in two hours. She was back to college on the Monday, and had no chronic 'drawn-out' illness at all. This was due to the fact that her fever had risen to 40°C (104°F) for four days prior to the i.v. vitamin C. Hers was a prime example of what can be done by natural methods.

(Glandular fever almost invariably leaves behind what is called 'post-viral' illness. This can last for months or even years. It sometimes lays the foundation for Chronic Fatigue and other illnesses later in life).

Nursing your child through natural infections

Although the natural measles infection is 'a good thing' (for an otherwise healthy child), it can be most uncomfortable. Your role then, is to nurse and comfort the child.

From the beginning, keep the child away from bright light – mostly they are photophobic (light sensitive). That is why these sick children welcome a quiet and darkened room in which to fight their little battle. But do NOT try to suppress the fever (see Fever Chapter).

Of course, your role will have begun months before, in providing good nutrition, plenty of fresh food, water and extra vitamin C[26] (1000 –2000 mg daily) and beta-carotene foods (the yellow and green foods), even some extra Vitamin A supplement. But also, zinc and magnesium. And a tight control of sugary foods. Sugar can lower white cell response by 50%. But no harm will come to a well nutritioned, vitamin C loaded child from naturally acquired measles. All creatures except humans (and one or two others) are able to manufacture ascorbic acid (Vit C). All animals use ascorbic acid to fight disease. A sick goat for instance, increases vitamin C production hundreds of times higher when sick than when well. What does that tell us?

However, if for some reason you become concerned, for instance, if the cough turns really bad and appears to affect the lungs, then call the doctor.

One important measure you can take to minimise lung and bronchial problems is to give the child the warm bath with Epsom salts we have mentioned. This will also 'draw-out' the rash, and in fact that is why it minimises the internal problems. It is very doubtful, if following the above instructions, that respiratory problems will commence.

You may ask, "Why do the authorities insist measles is dangerous and blinds or kills millions?"

This is certainly true in Third World countries, where nutrition is often very poor. But the London School of Tropical Health, in public statements of the past, has pointed out that given good nutrition this would not happen. Even in the Western world, half of the very few fatalities occur in persons with serious chronic disease or disability.[27]

A junk food diet of cheese, crackers, soda, cookies, chocolate and water – along with no fruit and vegetables whatsoever – caused a young college student to develop scurvy, a condition brought on by vitamin C deficiency.

Scurvy, which once affected sailors who did not get enough vitamin C in their diets, is characterized by symptoms such as bleeding gums, loose teeth, muscle degeneration and weakness. Another sign of scurvy is a change in skin colour on the legs, which results from bleeding underneath the skin. The student went to the doctor because he was experiencing swelling and bruising on his legs. He was also found to have bleeding gums and a rapid heartbeat.

Although the student was eating enough calories, researchers estimated that his vitamin C intake was about 0.1 milligram per day – well below the 90 milligrams per day recommended daily allowance (RDA) for non-smoking men (and many experienced physicians believe this to be a ridiculously low amount, barely above the scurvy level for some). His blood level of vitamin C was found to be at least four-fold below normal range.

He was advised to take a multivitamin and a vitamin C supplement, and after four days of use his symptoms greatly improved. The condition improved further after an additional two weeks of extra vitamin C.

Researchers stressed that people need vitamin C every day, and even though they may be eating enough food, they may not be getting enough vitamin C.

Scurvy or pre-scurvy occurs more often among the elderly and alcoholics, who often have unbalanced diets. But can be found in children and infants on poor diets and with mothers also on low vitamin C intake.

It must be remembered that today we live in an environment where our air, water and food is constantly contaminated with toxins and oxidants. To stay healthy in such a modern world we need a good deal more of many immune nutrients (like vitamin C) than is contained in the RDA's. Also, some people need more than others. An athlete in hard training needs many times more nutrients of all kinds than a sedentary person. And the same can be said for many occupations and circumstances (pregnancy for instance).

Contrasting a natural infection with vaccination

Having discussed what takes place in a normal ('wild') infection of measles, now contrast that with what happens when a child is vaccinated. Suddenly, without warning the immune system is beset by not one but three or even four simulated and concentrated viral attacks. And not through the mucus membranes, where defences are strong. But straight into the bloodstream.

Not only is this an attack which the body finds hard to handle, it is engaged with three or four viral challenges at once. Whereas, in nature, a child never has three viruses active at the same time.

But, there's more. This attack is accompanied by Axis powers totally strange to the body. Mercury, aluminium, formaldehyde, anti-freeze (some of the chemicals used in vaccines) can arrive at the same time!

The child's immune system is inclined to be overpowered by this array, and can usually only manage a short-term response (see below). Compare this list of poor, half-hearted responses to the full-blown healthy response of a typical wild measles infection described above.

Measles	about 10% have short fever or inflammation. Only 1% develops a rash
Mumps	only 1 in 100 develop swollen glands

The Diptheria, Tetanus and Pertussis 'triple antigen' shot produce more serious unnatural reactions. One in ten children can develop high-pitched unusual screaming (this figure varies down to one in one thousand – but is a common occurrence). There are other more serious reactions, including relapse into permanent brain damage and sometimes death (labelled SIDS).[28,29]

None of these fevers etc. last long enough to show a proper and orderly immune response.

As Dr Incao puts it: "If we now return to the original question of the mechanism of action of vaccinations, we find what I believe is the key to the puzzle. A vaccination consists of introducing a disease agent or disease antigen into an individual's body without causing the disease. If the disease agent provoked the whole immune system into action it would cause all the symptoms of the disease! The symptoms of a disease are primarily the symptoms (fever, pain, malaise, loss of function) of the acute inflammatory response to the disease."

No wonder the children's immune systems have become over-stimulated and auto-immune disease widespread.[30] Yet, there are immunologists who claim that a child can take 10,000 vaccines at once!

These were some of the reasons why Dr Incao was invited to speak to the US Senate Sub-Committee hearing on vaccine damage: "A critical point which is never mentioned by those advocating mandatory vaccination of children is that children's health has declined significantly since 1960 when vaccines began to be widely used. According to the National Health Interview Survey conducted annually by the National Centre for Health Statistics since 1957, a shocking 31% of US children today have a chronic health problem, 18% of children require special health care or related services and 6.7% of children have a significant disability due to a chronic physical or mental condition. Respiratory allergies, asthma and learning disabilities are the most common of these."

The vaccine problem of long term immunity

Not only is vaccine immunity questionable because of its side-effects, it also questionable because of its lack of long-term efficiency. One of the problems lies in the ability of virus to mutate or change their coats, so they can no longer be recognised.

For instance, influenza vaccination is foiled by viral mutation. Surface protein mutation allows influenza to persist in the human population by evading herd immunity. This process is termed 'antigenic drift'. (Jeffery Stuart, Los Alamos National Laboratory). Therefore the annual 'flu shot is a myth. A dangerous myth, because taking it annually brings you an annual dose of 50 mcg of mercury! Flu vaccines are still preserved with Hg (2003). And mercury can be accumulative.

Another problem is the validity of using antibodies as a measure of a successful immunisation. Anti-bodies are specialised proteins produced by the body defences that recognise a specific enemy (you may know them as IgM, IgG etc.). They bind onto the invader and make it easier to kill with leucocytes. When there are many antibodies then the immunisation is said to be 'good'. So goes the theory.

But, in *The New Scientist* (May 27, 2000) two scientists in AIDS research pointed out that "the assumption that successful vaccines work by simply producing antibodies is almost certainly wrong."

The scientists described how a vaccine for a virus in horses was successful in inducing antibodies against the virus, but the vaccinated horses died faster than the unvaccinated ones. The researcher commented that, "We are ignorant as to why these vaccinated horses died, even with high antibodies. It's an issue people haven't wanted to think about, but we might have to."

Measles & mumps antibodies found before immunisation

With these question marks around, we have to ask why vaccinate at all and risk the danger when a Danish study of non-vaccinated young people found nearly all were already naturally immune to measles (99%) and mumps (80%).[31]

Are antibodies really always workers or just markers?

The American paediatrician researcher Dr Philip Incao put it this way: "Vaccine science and practice have always been based on certain assumptions, which we are only now beginning to be examined. One of these is that antibodies in the blood (humoral immunity) confer protection against illness, and that the level correlates with the degree of protection. This apparent protection has been observed for decades in many types of diseases. *It is not known however whether the antibodies persisting in the blood for months or years after an infectious disease* ***are themselves responsible*** *for protecting us from recurrences of that disease or* ***whether they are sometimes merely markers*** *of a protection accomplished by another part of the immune system."* Evidence of this problem lies in the fact that often in vaccinated populations, with high antibody levels, the disease to which they are supposed to be immune becomes an epidemic. Maybe this is why the authorities say an unvaccinated child is a 'risk' to unvaccinated children. If the vaccine was so safe, why should the *vaccinated* child be at risk!

Modern science has discovered a dazzling array and myriad complexities involved in the immune system. It is now known that the interrelationships are far more puzzling than any computer driven 'flow-chart' could, at this point, fully explain.

It is best for us to support this wonderful inbuilt mechanism we call our immune system, but not to interfere with it otherwise.

CHAPTER THIRTEEN

A word on fevers in your child

Myths and facts about fevers

"Fevers in childhood are common. They signify that a child is experiencing and fighting an inflammatory condition, usually an infection. The fever is not in itself a disease, but rather a helpful natural biologic mechanism for combating the disease. Fever need not be feared nor treated medicinally but for exceptional circumstances."

Princeton Paediatricians Mark B. Levin, MD
and Timothy Patrick-Miller, MD

'Normal' fevers are the immune system at work. They defend the body against disease. Never stop a good man when he is working! (Examples of abnormal fevers are given below.)

If your child becomes infected by disease-producing microbes a fever should develop. These microbes often produce proteins called *pyrogens* that cause your child's thermostat (heat controller, the hypothalamus) to reset upwards. Now the body begins to overheat. This is really bad news for the pathogens, because they will die at far less a temperature than the cells of your child's body. In fact, your child could withstand a temperature of 42.2°C (107.96°F) before brain cells began to wither. Even cancer cells die at 42°C (107.6°F), if the temperature is maintained long enough.

Humans die when body temperature reaches about 44.5°C (112°F). But super-low temperatures are also dangerous – below 24.5°C is close to fatal.

Fevers in children used to be regarded as normal events by our wise forebears. They were not suppressed. In fact, one sign of a weak immune system is that no fever is produced in a common infectious disease.

Here are some modern myths about fevers.

Myth 1 Fevers keep on going up if unchecked
Truth Unless a child is in a hot place, or overdressed the brains thermostat will stop the fever at 40.5°C (105°F). Even viral

and bacterial infections normally stop at 40.5 °C. However, the fever should stop inside three days. An example of this built-in safety mechanism is the case of scarlet fever, once a common disease for children, but now rare. Here is a 100-year old description from a rare antique book in my library by Dr Leslie Mackenzie MA MD, then the Medical Member of the Local Government Board for Scotland and Medical Inspector of School Children:

"Here is a school child of ten, just admitted. His face is flushed and there is no rash on it. His hands, arms and lower limbs, however, all show a bright red eruption – the rash of scarlet fever. His pulse runs at a high rate. His temperature has gone up to 103 °F or 104 °F (39.4 °C or 40 °C). It will remain there for a day or two. The rash will fade away in 48 hours ... in perhaps four days he will be, apparently, back to his normal state."

The good doctor never mentioned trying to reduce the fever in his Chapter on fevers. It was a given that fevers completed their natural course. Of course, parents are concerned (as we were once, when our daughter had a 40 °C fever plus some mild delirium for four days), but must learn to relax – the 'body is the Hero' and knows best! It certainly helps you to relax when you know that a fever is a 'good thing' and not a 'bad thing'.[81]

However, poisoning, exposure to toxic substances, or heatstroke *are* dangerous elevators of temperature. Heatstroke usually occurs as a result of too much sunshine on a hot day. The ambient temperature (the surrounding air) is so hot that the body cannot cool down through its usual mechanism of radiating the heat away from itself. If it is also humid, then evaporation won't work either.

Fevers are also not so good in the very young. If your child is less than two months old and has a fever of 38 °C (100 °F) or over, call your doctor.

Myth 2 Fevers damage the brain

Truth Fevers below 42.2 °C (108 °F) do not damage the brain. Even fevers of 40.5 ° are a normal result of a good immune response. Do not quell these fevers. Even if a chill develops, do not 'wrap her up' warmer. You are fighting against her immune defences. A chill is sign of a rising fever and the body taking steps to control it.

When the sweating begins this shows the fever is about to fall soon. It is the crisis point, a good sign that your child has mounted a successful defence. Fevers accompanied by other symptoms, such as constipation and vomiting for instance, extreme weakness or very rapid pulse or fevers rising fast can be signs of more difficult problems than a common childhood infection. (See Chapter 11).

Myth 3 Always give aspirin or similar for a fever

Truth According to a series of studies at the University of Maryland (1978–1987) quelling fevers with aspirin can actually prolong the illness. The University's Center for Vaccine Development found that flu sufferers who took one of the anti-fever medications were sick an average of 3.5 days longer than people who did not take either of the drugs. On average, flu symptoms lasted 5.3 days in participants who did not take aspirin or acetaminophen, compared with 8.8 days in people who took the anti-fever drugs.

Myth 4 37°C is 'normal'

Truth 37°C (98.6°F) is an average only. Temperatures vary through the day. Some children have a normal temperature of up to 37.4°C (99.4°F). Others maybe normal at 35.8°C (96.6°F). Paediatric doctors at Princeton University point out that the significance of a fever depends on the child and the circumstances – not the temperature. "The answer relates not to a number, but to the child's functional state and associated symptoms. If a child with an identified condition has a fever at any level and responds to social interaction in a manner that is appropriate for the child's developmental stage, then concern is lessened."[81]

Myth 5 Always use a rectal temperature or an ear thermometer.

Truth There is no need to risk a rectal perforation. Underarm (axillary) is fine. Do not put the thermometer in the ear. Dr Robert Mendlesohn, a famous old paediatrician, put it this way "Never place anything in the ear that is smaller than your elbow!" Ear thermometers are also notoriously inaccurate and inclined to read too high.

Points to watch

- No matter what the temperature, if your child experiences difficulty breathing, twitching, or repeated vomiting, or strange movements – or has other similar concerns, then call your doctor.
- If he is continuously listless, irritable, or appears seriously ill – call your doctor.
- Encourage your child to rest and make sure he eats properly. Maybe soups, or vegetable juices, but more solid food if he will take it. Give plenty to drink. Avoid all sugars.

CHAPTER FOURTEEN

How to treat common childhood illnesses

"The best doctors are Dr. Diet, Dr. Quiet and Dr. Merryman."

Jonathan Swift

This classic Chapter was written by the noted American paediatrician Dr Philip Incao MD and is gratefully used by permission.

All of the common illnesses of childhood are inflammations. 'Infection' is the wrong word for them because it suggests that we get sick because germs invade us. This is misleading. We are always exposed to and often harbour germs and yet we only occasionally get sick. Why do we get sick when we do?

In order to be healthy we must keep an inner balance in body and soul while all the time growing and changing from birth to death. Childhood is the time of most rapid growth and dramatic change, and a child will remodel and renew his body many times as he grows. Every remodelling job requires some demolition, a breaking down of part of the inherited bodily structure in order to rebuild it better. This breaking down of old cells and tissues results in debris, which must be cleaned up before the body rebuilds itself. *It is the immune system* which does the breaking down by causing cell death, and when necessary, fever and inflammation to destroy and digest foreign or outworn bodily material. *And it is the immune system* which cleans up the digested material and debris by pushing it out of the body. That is why children so often will have skin rashes and discharges of mucus or pus, *because their immune systems are actively working.* Debris that remains in the body may act like a poison, or may cause allergies or repeated inflammations later on. Germs do not 'attack' us, but they often multiply wherever the body's living substance is dying, breaking down, and being discharged. Germs don't cause illnesses: they feed on them.

Every childhood inflammation, every cold, sore throat, earache, fever and rash is a healing crisis and a cleansing process, a strong effort by the human spirit to remodel the body so it can be a more suitable dwelling. Natural and homeopathic remedies help and promote this cleansing process and help the illness to work its way *out* of the body in order for healing to occur. Antibiotics, aspirin, Tylenol, ibuprofen and other anti-inflammatory drugs cool down and suppress the 'fire' of the immune system so that the symptoms subside *before* the illness has fully worked its way out of the body. When an inflammation is suppressed in this way, and prevented from fully discharging its toxins, then either the inflammation will come back, or else the tendency to allergies and asthma will be increased. Recent research has confirmed that antibiotics and vaccinations are a cause of increased allergies and asthma.

It rarely happens in healthy people that the inflammatory response of the immune system may get out of control. In such cases an antibiotic may be needed. Although an antibiotic may be life-saving, it never heals an inflammation; it only suppresses it. The causes of the inflammation must still be healed after the antibiotic treatment, otherwise the immune system may remain weakened.

Cleansing and detox

In addition to any remedies you may use, *the first and best thing you should always do* at the onset of any inflammation, fever, cold or "infection" is to cleanse the body as follows:

1 Give infants a glycerine rectal suppository. For adults and children over one year of age, give a Bisacodyl (Dulcolax) suppository. If you prefer, an enema may be used instead of a suppository. (Of course, do not use any of these if diarrhea is present.) *After the initial suppository or enema, it is important to keep the cleansing going until the illness is all better by giving a dose of Milk of Magnesia once daily for 3–5 days.*

Children, 1–5 years of age	1–2 tablespoons or 2–4 tablets
Children, 5–12 years of age	2–3 tablespoons or 4–6 tablets
Over 12 and adults	4 tablespoons or 6-8 tablets

(After the first 3-5 days and until fever and pain are all gone, stewed prunes will help to keep bowels loose.)

Infants under one year	Fennel tea and diluted juices from stewed organic apricots and prunes will help to loosen the stools.

2 Drink lots of warm herb teas, especially horsetail (equisetum) which cleanses the kidneys.

3 **Strictly avoid all protein foods!** See under 'Diet' for further details.

Body warmth and fever

"We have lost the commonsense and the wisdom that used to prevail in the approach to childhood diseases. Too often, instead of reinforcing the organism's defences, fever and symptoms are relentlessly suppressed … this is not always without consequences. On the other hand, if a child's organism is affected deeply by a disease, as in measles – there can be positive consequences. For a child to defeat a disease by its own means enables it to mature its immune system and develop increased resistance."

(Group of Concerned Swiss Doctors, Berne, March 1990)

Children should always be warmly dressed for the weather. This will increase their body's ability to handle inflammations. The normal body temperature in a healthy child or adult should be generally speaking around 36.9 °C (98.5 °F). A somewhat higher temperature is better than a significantly sub-normal temperature, which indicates that not enough warmth is being produced by the body. Viruses and bacteria in us grow faster and toxins accumulate when the body temperature is lower and they are all cleared faster from the body by the immune system when the body temperature is higher. Weather permitting, young children should be dressed in natural fibers with 3 layers on top and 2 on bottom. Wool socks are very helpful to support a healthy body temperature. Children under 3 years especially should wear caps or hats to protect the body from warmth loss and the intensity of the sun.

Fever should not be regarded as a dangerous or unhealthy process in the body. It is actually the body's messenger and a healthy response to the presence of something foreign or toxic that the body needs to get rid of. If we feel very uncomfortable, achy or even delirious with fever, these are symptoms caused by the toxicity, the poisons, in our system. The fever isn't the problem, it's part of the solution! Giving Tylenol or Advil for a fever is like killing the messenger.

Many parents have a dread of fevers because they expect them to lead to convulsions or brain damage. *This is simply not true!* The great majority of fevers are perfectly benign, and the great majority of children are not susceptible to fever convulsions and don't get them even with very high fevers. Fever convulsions happen only in a small minority of children who are so constituted as to have a low threshold for convulsions. Even in these susceptible children fever convulsions are rare events, usually happening only once or twice between 6 months and 6 years of age.

Fever convulsions do not cause any permanent damage to the brain or nervous system.

- Lowering a fever with Tylenol, baths or anything else will *not* prevent convulsions.
- The minority of children who are susceptible to fever convulsions will outgrow their susceptibility after age 7.
- *A fever convulsion is much less likely to occur* if the recommendations in these pages for bowel cleansing, diet, quiet and warmth are promptly followed at the first sign of illness in children, as well as giving the appropriate natural or homeopathic remedies.

It is the *toxicity* from certain diseases and certain immunizations which may rarely cause brain damage or convulsions in children or adults, regardless of whether the fever is high or low. But *fever itself*, even when 40°C (104° F) or over, will *not* cause brain damage. In the very rare case when a fever goes over 41°C (106°F), you should call your doctor.

Therefore, when a child has a fever, dress him even *more warmly* than usual with layers of cotton or wool. Keep the patient warm enough that the cheeks are red and the hands and feet are warm, but there is no sweat or perspiration. The body in its wisdom wants and needs to be hot in order to burn out the illness. When the fever is rising, we feel chilled and want to get warm under blankets. When the fever breaks and then starts to come down, only then do we feel hot and sweat and throw off the blankets. This is the natural way the immune system burns out the illness and discharges its toxins.

It is best *not* to give aspirin, or Tylenol, ibuprofen or baths for a fever. There is no evidence whatsoever that these prevent fever convulsions. In fact, recent research suggests that *fever-lowering drugs may actually be harmful by suppressing the immune system and increasing the body's retention of toxicity, thus making complications and prolongation of the illness more likely.*

Don't forget, fever drives the toxins out of the body. Tylenol and other fever-reducing drugs can therefore make us more toxic! This explains why, in some viral inflammations of children, aspirin increases the risk of Reye Syndrome, and ibuprofen seems to increase the risk of serious bacterial complications. Tylenol is likely to do the same, as well as having a well-known toxic effect on the liver, which can be very dangerous at higher doses.

Healing occurs when our toxins have been fully digested and discharged from the body. Traditional medical wisdom has always recognized that the discharge of pus, mucus or rash is a *healing response* to the underlying illness.

If a child or adult with a high fever is very uncomfortable and restless, this is a sign of toxicity and the previously mentioned cleansing measures are needed. You may also rub the arms and legs and head with a washcloth moistened with tepid water and Arnica tincture or lemon juice. (From the neck to the knees the child should not be undressed.) Rub vigorously to make the skin red and this will help to dissipate excess body heat through the skin. *This restlessness and irritability during a fever are caused by circulating toxins in the body and can often be prevented by following the directions under "Cleansing and Detox".*

Diet

When someone has, or is coming down with any type of inflammation, cold or fever, the diet should be restricted. When your body is trying to digest and eliminate toxic substances it will help if you don't have to digest much food at the same time. Therefore, the general rule is to **avoid protein foods** during the acute illness. These are: meat, eggs, dairy, nuts, fish and legumes (beans, peas, lentils, soy, etc.).

The sick person should have a mainly liquid diet of vegetable broth, herb teas and fruit juices, but no juices colder than room temperature. Fruit, cooked vegetables, grains, and light crackers are also suitable.

Another general rule is that when sick, eating *less* is better than eating more. If the patient is not hungry then she is better off not eating. On the other hand, when your patient in the middle of her illness is suddenly hungry, then let her eat light, non-protein food and she will be quickly satisfied. Add protein only when you are *sure* the illness is really over.

The return of appetite is a sign of getting over the illness, but those first meals after the fever is gone should be light ones. Don't be too eager to have your child regain the lost weight; this will happen soon enough quite naturally as your child's appetite and strength return. After the illness, reintroduce the restricted foods gradually and carefully.

Quiet

Most adults have experienced how, during a fever or any inflammatory illness, we crave peace and quiet and are disturbed by noises and sounds which usually don't bother us when we are well. Children have this same need for peace and quiet during their illnesses, though they will rarely express it. Instead, out of boredom they will ask to listen to the radio, tapes or watch TV. These kinds of stimulation are best avoided, especially for younger children, and should be replaced by just 'being there' for your child during his or her illness in a peaceful, unhurried and reassuring way. Keep them quietly under covers in bed or on a couch away from the hustle and bustle of household activity. *The more they can sleep during an illness, the better.*

Illness is a time to remove oneself from the usual pressures and routines of life and to 'veg out' totally and to allow ones body to repair and renew itself in the context of a peaceful and supportive environment. Very often illness can provide a wonderful opportunity for renewed communication and bonding between parent and child.

CHAPTER FIFTEEN

Encouragement for parents who seek God for help

"Therapies for depression and anxiety that incorporate religious beliefs in treatment result in faster recovery from illness than do traditional therapies."

Harold Koenig MD
Associate Professor of Psychiatry
Center for the Study of Religion/Spirituality and Health
Duke University USA

I find that many desperate mothers and fathers have sought God in prayer to find a way to help their child with ASD. And many times their prayer has been answered in terms of finding good natural resources and people who can help them. Some of their stories are given later in this Chapter.

In his book, *The Faith Factor: proof of the healing power of prayer*, Georgetown University medical professor Dale Matthews says, "Scientific studies show that faith involvement helps people prevent illness, recover from illness, and – most remarkably – live longer. The more religiously committed you are, the more likely you are to benefit."

One practical example of these benefits was found in a study of hospitalised patients.

- Hospital stays are nearly 2½ times longer for older patients who don't have a religious affiliation (1997).
- Heart-surgery patients assigned chaplain intervention showed an average two days shorter length of stay, or about $4,200 cost savings per patient (1995).

Summation of physical- and mental-health studies, Harold Koenig MD

An interesting personal story comes from American hospital midwife-nurse, Ginny Weisz:

> "Ginny recounts a vivid incident a few years ago, when a baby's heart stopped beating during birth. As the medical team worked for more than 30 minutes to revive the infant, Ms. Weisz prayed intensely.

> Suddenly she said firmly out loud, "Father, let this baby live." And, she added, "I believed He would." The baby revived and turned out to be a perfectly normal child. Weisz has three children and a busy life as a practicing nurse, but she is now considering going back to school to get her PhD in nursing so she can research the effects of prayer on health.
>
> *Christian Science Monitor, 2003*

One word of caution is necessary on such experiences as Ginny Weisz. If a totally dedicated mother prays such a prayer and normal life is *not* restored to her child, then this can have as devastating effect, equal but opposite to the joy of an obviously answered prayer. The person feels unworthy, or can lose faith entirely and become more depressed than before.

One real answer is this: in the experience of very many, a loving God has purposes which we cannot fathom while in this world. But always, in answer to serious prayer from the heart He gives a certain peace to bear our load, and often He will also lead the enquirer (if willing) to a natural source of healing, using the methods – for instance, as found in this book or similar. Several thousand of stories like this can be found in the work of Dr George Malkmus, a prominent and successful American minister who was cured of bowel cancer through natural methods in 1976. In gratitude to God he started a health retreat that began to cure thousands through natural, mostly dietary methods. Today he has over 1.2 million people who follow his programs.[62]

Dr Malkmus first came to realise that God likes to do His miracles through natural laws, after he had seen several of his ministerial friends die of cancer despite the earnest prayers of many friends, congregations and fellow ministers. During his own advancing cancer, he began to look for alternative methods and was led to a natural health centre in Florida.

Every scientific discovery reveals more questions to be answered

It is a fact that in our work of restoring body function, and thus immune system dynamics, we are using natural methods to enhance the masterpiece of Creation we call our bodies. As science advances and more and more knowledge is obtained on exactly how this masterpiece functions, the more intelligent can be our co-operation.

Make no mistake, the best scientists – as the Nobel Prize winners who 'discover' bits like the RNA/DNA puzzle, are only *discovering* what is already there! Like a small boy with a new toy, they take it to pieces to see how it works. But they are not the ToyMaker. And even now, in the year 2003 – after thousands of years of investigation, there are important 'bits' and functions in the body that are still not fully understood. For instance, the genome make-up (in the study of genes) has advanced to the stage where a new horizon has taken over – which is beyond genes themselves. It is now found that genes are controlled by a sub-strat that is dynamic. They are influenced by even smaller entities in constant flux. This dynamism is equally as important as the genes! The genes are merely a framework for another world to be explored! Yet these 'junk genes', as they were called a few years ago, were considered just that – junk! They appeared to have no coding function. The mystery of life deepens – not simplifies, with each passing year.

Even the atheistic evolutionist Richard Dawkins (an Oxford scientist) says, "There is enough information capacity in a single human cell to store the *Encyclopaedia Britannica*, all 30 volumes, three or four times over."

We can only just begin to comprehend and bit by bit find out the secrets and purposes of God, the Maker of this complexity. But for many parents who pray in faith because they feel the need, the reality of a God Who listens is sometimes shown in unexpected ways.

I gave an example of this earlier in the book – a mother prayed earnestly one morning that God would lead her to someone who could help her ASD son. She sat next to a woman on the train who knew of our Clinic's work with children, even though she lives 600km away. We were able to reverse that child's problems.

In our small group meetings every Tuesday evening is a hospital radiology nurse, Laurel. She told us of the problems she was experiencing with her 15-month old daughter's health. So, we all prayed for her to find an answer.

The next week it so happened that only Laurel and her husband turned up. It was the 'flu season! Six of the ten were away. I was able to question her about the little girl. The evening turned into a clinic session! I was told that the little girl could not sleep through the night and was exhausting the parents. The symptoms were very similar to the early onset of vaccine damage to the gut. I mentioned the leaky gut, and it was obvious even in such a young one. The parents were very interested (I had previously helped her repair a wrist damaged at the hospital months before, and not healing).

A week later, Laurel told me that she spoke about her baby to the Hospital paediatrician. She mentioned the bowel problems but did not say the words 'leaky gut'. The doctor thought for a moment, and said off-handedly, as if to himself, "Hmm, maybe a leaky gut?". So, both she and I were surprised that this probable diagnosis came from two such different sources.

We treated that infant with total sugar-free and dairy-free diet, bowel flora, 4-Life Transfer Factor and RejuvenX gut wall repair. By next small group time, the baby was sleeping through the night and 'heaps better' according to her mother!

We both acknowledged that the Providence of God had made this possible. Without the absentees at that previous meeting, we would have had little time and she would have had no inclination to discuss her child.

Experiences like these among medical professionals and others are part of a world-wide shift in focus – more advanced than you would think – that is encouraging a return to the faith that once guided the great majority of people in their plans and daily living.

Three recently (2003) published studies showed:

- Patients are 12 times more likely to survive open-heart surgery if they depend on their religious faith and social support.
- Over a 28-year study period, mortality for frequent attendees of religious services was almost 25 percent lower than for people who attended less frequently. For women, the figure was 35 percent.
- Those who attend religious services at least once a week have been shown to have stronger immune system functioning.

In recently discussing spirituality and medical outcomes, David Larson of the National Institute for Healthcare Research (NIHR) called the power of faith 'the forgotten factor'. He says it has been neglected and mishandled, because of scientific attitudes toward religion.

Many parents of hurting children say they have found peace and strength in daily communion with God. I understand what they say, for this book and my own life has been enriched by such faith meetings with God, who we can know as Saviour and Friend and Guide to help us find truth in healing procedures. These parents will find a free and daily useful resource to help faith grow, at the website prayer@childrenofdestiny.org.

This provides a daily encouragement to those who have ASD children and email facilities. It is run by two parents whose son Nicholas was diagnosed with autism in 2001.

Jack and Rebecca Sytsema are both ordained Christian ministers who have been involved in international prayer ministry for the past 10 years. Jack is the accountant for the Autism Education Action Group, a local secular group dedicated to furthering awareness of and interventions for autism in Colorado. Rebecca currently serves as Associate Publisher and CEO of Wagner Publications, a Christian publishing house. She has co-authored six Christian books to date. She also sits on the Board of Directors for the Autism Education Action Group. She works from home where "she is first and foremost mom to Nicholas and Samuel, a neuro-typical toddler". Rebecca writes:

> "We believe in the power of prayer and believe that God's hand is firmly on Nicholas' life. We have implemented several other interventions for Nicholas, including the gluten- and casein-free diet, several biomedical interventions, and an intensive program of Applied Behaviour Analysis. While each intervention has helped Nicholas come to new levels of success, we firmly hold to the belief that the most powerful intervention we have brought into our son's life has been to give him over to God and allow Him to order our steps concerning Nicholas. Although the path has been a difficult one, we have seen steady progress as God works new miracles day by day. God has yet to disappoint us in any area with which we have fully trusted Him!"

CHAPTER SIXTEEN

Without mercy or morals

What pharmaceuticals are doing to our children

"One cannot necessarily trust the government doctors."

Dr Richard Nicholson
Editor, *Bulletin of Medical Ethics*, Jan 1996

"Billions are spent devising ways to alter criteria until the outcome is what the pharmaco wants, and a double blind placebo controlled study can be pointed in any direction desired. I no longer trust any of these studies. I see nothing but intentional deception."

Personal communication from
an experienced practicing psychiatrist

Mind altering medical drugs are now being used on children around the world in ever increasing numbers. A medical journal has shown that prescription of psyche drugs for children doubled in the 1990's and today almost matches adult usage (*Archives of Pediatrics & Adolescent Medicine,* 2003). These psychiatric drugs have side-effects. As the founder of the huge drug company Eli Lilly once said, "If it doesn't have side effects, then it isn't a drug". These side effects include death, suicidal tendencies and damage that can sometimes be worse than death, plus lesser but life-altering events. Some of these are comparatively rare, but not rare for those who are on the receiving end. In total they affect tens of thousands. For parents the worst aspects of these problems are these:

- parents are usually not told of them;
- some are not even licensed for under 18 year olds (e.g. Paxil);
- the damaged victims are ignored, and any link with their drug is denied;
- compensation requires huge effort, many years and great cost;
- more and more are available without prescription;
- the now widespread advertising handles the truth lightly;
- side effects (so-called adverse reactions) are seldom recorded;
- the worst side-effect is long-term addiction leading to a ruined life;

- some package warnings tell patient he must continue taking the drug (risperdone); and
- so good is this for drug companies that they are designing implants for their 'hooked' customers

Let us look more closely at an example of what goes on behind the scenes.

Paxil – a story of deaths and deceit

Taken off the market in Ireland

Also known overseas as Seroxat, Paxil has been prescribed for children with ASD problems, even though it is specifically not recommended for those under 18. Why not? Because Paxil has caused suicidal impulses and multiple claims of suicidal deaths in young people. The drug company (GlaxoSmithKline) was aware of the possibility of these incidents. On October 12, 2002 the Irish Department of Medicines took Seroxat off the market. The manufacturer, GlaxoSmithKline, had failed to adequately warn patients about possible suicidal behaviour when using Seroxat. (See http://paxilsupport.homestead.com for stories of mothers who lost their children).

Yet, after years of lobbying and media attention, it was not until June 10 2003 that the British Department of Health issued this warning:

> "'New expert advice recommends that the drug Seroxat (paroxetine) is not used to treat children and teenagers under the age of 18 years, for depressive illness,' said Professor Alasdair Breckenridge, Chairman of the Medicines and Healthcare products Regulatory Agency.
>
> New data, received within the last two weeks, has been evaluated and considered by the Committee on Safety of Medicines, (CSM) and its Expert Working Group on SSRIs. It shows that there is an increase in the rate of self harm and potentially suicidal behaviour in this age group, when Seroxat is used for depressive illness. It has become clear that the benefits of Seroxat in children for the treatment of depressive illness do not outweigh these risks."

In America, the *New York Times* (August 2003) said that:

> "... doctors are just beginning to react to the finding – reported first by British drug authorities in June and then endorsed the next

week by the Food and Drug Administration – that unpublished studies about Paxil show that it carries a substantial risk of prompting teenagers and children to consider suicide.

Because the studies also found that Paxil was no more effective than a placebo in treating young people's depression, the regulators recommended that doctors write no new Paxil prescriptions for patients under 18. Experts say that the suicide risk is highest in the first few weeks young patients are on the drug."

The drug had previously been widely prescribed for children by doctors using their discretion, which had been allowable. The problem is that the average doctor often is not informed of what is occurring after a drug is prescribed, let alone what is happening in the wider world.

Children on ADD drugs – 160 recorded deaths

The Class Actions against psychiatrists & drug companies

Year 2000 estimates of the number of children diagnosed with symptoms of ADD and ADHD in USA varied from 5–7 million (10–15% of children), who filled 11 million methylphenidate (Ritalin) prescriptions in 1999. A steep increase since 500,000 'diagnosed' cases in 1985. The epidemic rages on, doubling every 3–4 years.

Methylphenidate is a stimulant of the amphetamine ('speed') family and shares the same abuse potential as the amphetamines – which paradoxically counteracts abnormal hyperactivity, the very symptom it produces. It is produced by Novartis of Switzerland (formerly Ciba-Geigy) and is the most used drug of several similar chemicals.

In Australia, second only to the USA in usage of the Ritalin-type drugs, the pattern is being mirror imaged, with some 10–15% of children believed to suffer from the problems.

In Great Britain, where the Government is among world-wide dissenters questioning the popularity of Ritalin (it is not, after all, a British company from which taxes can be earned) 'only' 157,000 prescriptions were sold in 1999, although that represented a 25% increase from 1998.

While the Ritalin-type drugs undoubtably restore a degree of normalcy in attention span, concentration and therefore of learning ability and have changed the lives of many ADD affected children and adults, they are a crutch only. There is no cure effected by using them because the causes are not addressed (they have the same stimulating effect on non-ADD brains). Moreover, as we shall see, there are many known side effects and sometimes a terrible price to pay. On the other hand, there are non-invasive, gentle methods that also restore normalcy but **without** side-effects. It is the typical history of the repression of these facts that concerned the first part of this book. The rest of the book presents what I and many other biological practitioners have found to be actual ways of curing the problem.

Since most if not all of the information, statistics, treatment and understanding of these childhood behavioural disorders (CBD's) come to us from the USA this Chapter looks at the current trends and the politico-legal battle now raging in North America, where six class actions have been filed. Unless we think and choose for ourselves this history is destined, it would seem, to unfortunately but inevitably be repeated in Australia – part of the 'McDonalding' of our nation. But this time it is serious, really serious. Children are dying from the drugs. According to Dr Fred Baughman Jr, a vocal whistle-blower in the Ritalin-War in America, the FDA's Division of Pharmacology lists 2,993 adverse reactions between 1990 and 1997. These include 160 deaths and 569 hospitalizations of which 36 were life-threatening. Imagine, 160 families bereaving a child from a behavioural disorder drug causing death. How many Australian families have been told this possibility when prescribed Ritalin? So far, I have found no one who knows. The saddest part is that there are simple ways to fix ADHD without drugs, as you have read in this book.

One of the deaths attributed to Ritalin by Baughman, a consulting neurologist, was featured on the CBS *Hard Copy* program on June 24, 1998. It is a heart-breaking tale. CBS told the story of twelve-year old Stephanie Hall of Canton in Idaho, 'a lovely, healthy, normal girl' (apart from ear infections – see Chapter 3) with a great love of books and of her friends. 'Stephie' was observed by her first grade teacher to lack some concentration and was making 'noises'. The teacher suggested to Stephie's mother Janet, that she be tested for ADD and to see the school psychologist at no cost. Stephie was duly diagnosed with ADD and prescribed Ritalin. Then her headaches began – everyday except on week-ends when she did not use Ritalin. Despite Stephie taking the drug, her teacher continued to complain about her behaviour and Stephie's Ritalin dose was increased (together with some behaviour modification approaches). Over the next five years the dose increased from 5mg morning and noon until it reached 40mg daily. Her behaviour and school performance improved, but disturbing symptoms developed. During Ritalin usage times she developed nausea and stomach aches and the headaches worsened. Mood swings and bizarre behaviour appeared. Her neurologist noticed incoordination.

One day in fourth grade, to the horror of day-care workers at the centre she attended after school, Stephanie suddenly took off and raced across a busy five-lane highway. They called her desperately, but she yelled back at them, "I am 10 years old now" and kept running, narrowly avoiding a terrible accident. Because of this, her mother had to cease work during after-school hours.

One day in the Summer break Stephie suddenly 'zoned out' and seemed disconnected. She said to her mother, "I love you" (which words they often shared), but then she said it again and this time her face held an empty stare.

Then Stephie said, "I see her again."

"Who?" asked Janet.

"The angel – she looks mad."

Then Stephie snapped out of her illusion and described to her mother that she saw angels with four wings and some were red and some were blue.

Janet said that the incident reminded her of the first times Stephie took Ritalin and saw angels.

In that last year of her life, Stephie showed herself to be friendly and 'a good girl', making friends easily and deciding on a career as a paramedic. Then suddenly, her behaviour changed in fits of swearing and anger. Later that year, Janet became so concerned she asked the paediatrician to increase the Ritalin. The doctor agreed and increased drug dose to 25mg in the morning and 15mg in the afternoon.

The next morning after the increased dose began, Stephie's father went to wake her for school. She did not respond. The shocked paramedics found her cold and dead.

Coronary finding: Death from natural causes – cardiac arrhythmia.

Janet called in Dr Baughman to review the case. The neurologist pointed out that this finding concludes that all diseases or abnormalities, such as Ritalin, which could contribute to such a death have been ruled out. He asked the question, "How often do normal, disease-free and drug-free 12-year old's develop a cardiac arrhythmia and die suddenly – with no family history?"

The coroner apparently never considered Ritalin to have been the cause of Stephie's death, despite the fact that the FDA Pharmacovigilance Unit has recorded 160 deaths from the drug. Or, the fact that Stephanie's dosage was almost always in the 1.0–1.6 mg/kg of bodyweight range, which is higher than the recommended range for children of her weight (0.3–0.6 mg/kg).

Furthermore, the coroner may have been unaware that acute episodes of hallucination early in therapy can point to toxic or abnormal reaction to the drug (Lucas and Weiss,1971 – cited in medical texts).

Moreover, Ritalin is known to cause palpitations, cardiac arrhythmia, tachycardia and hypertension. Ritalin can also cause problems in the heart muscle itself (Fisher, 1972). Fisher did this work on an adult who had been taking Ritalin for 4½ years. He found abnormal membranes accumulated in the heart muscle. In 1994, Fisher working with fellow researcher Henderson, once again proved his findings. They exposed experimental mice and rats to methylphenidate (MP) and found identical excess membranes under the electron microscope to those seen in the adult human heart in 1972. The researchers have shown that MP and other amphetamine-like drugs interfere with normal phospholipid (fat) chemistry.

Other alternative drugs to Ritalin with similar molecular structure, such as desipramine – a tricyclic antidepressant – can also cause severe side-effects, sometimes leading to cardiac death (16 deaths in America among children with ADHD). Another drug, pemoline, said to be the safest of the stimulants, caused 13 cases of liver failure leading to death or liver transplant up to May, 1996.

Reading, 'riting, 'rithmatic and Ritalin

The childhood industry

In 1980, the name Attention Deficit Disorder was coined by the American Psychiatric Association (APA) to identify a syndrome (a group of symptoms) affecting the learning and behaviour of American school children. Although no actual apparent physiological disease mechanism had been found (which is still the case, according to the Establishment) a disease had been 'named'. The next step was commercialisation of this new disease.

Teaming up with Ciba-Geigy (now Novartis), the manufacturers of Ritalin, the APA organised a support group called CHADD (Children & Adults with Attention Deficit Disorder). CHADD worked closely with the US Department of Education and was financed by Ciba-Geigy to the tune of cash grants of $900,000 plus in-kind services.

Although this intimate tie between educators and selected parents may at first sound a reasonable way to find an answer to a problem, its connection and financing from a single commercial entity (with but one aim) is the beginnings of corruption and when linked to an authoritarian stance on behalf of a potentially dangerous drug must be considered a major assault on the freedom and health of American school children. This was shown to be fact by Public Broadcasting Service (PBS) investigative journalists in 1995–96. They found that in 1994, the US Department of Education, under contract HS92017001 gave funding for a Washington Institute to produce two videos on ADD, both starring film actors. Parts of the videos sounded like an infomercial for Ritalin.

In 1996, PBS interviewed a Department of Education spokesman. He was asked if he was aware that the parents who spoke so enthusiastically about Ritalin on the videos were Board members of CHADD? And did he know that CHADD had received cash grants of $900,000 plus services from Ciba-Geigy? Obviously embarrassed the bureaucrat denied all such knowledge. (Exactly how much knowledge the proponents of Ritalin have regarding its side effects is also unclear. That year, a CHADD spokesperson said she had never heard of the Stephie Hall case described above. If their information is fed by the drug maker, then – like the chicken that lays an egg – what you get depends on the feed.)

The executive producer of the documentary, John Merrow, reported that Ritalin had become so plentiful that a black market had developed on the school playground. Ritalin can be crushed and snorted for a cheap buzz.

This revelation was followed in the year 2000 by a series of class actions against Novartis and the APA. The lawsuits, lodged in New Jersey and California, follow a third class action filed in Texas in May, **alleging that Novartis conspired with the APA to promote the diagnosis of ADHD and fuel the market for Ritalin.**

Four years earlier, in 1996, the World Health Organisation warned that Ritalin over-use had reached dangerous proportions.

Australia beware! Some 2-year old toddlers now on psyche drugs

On 21 August, 2000 the *Newcastle Herald* reported that:

> "At least 800 Hunter children are being prescribed psychotropic drugs despite little evidence the practice is safe or effective, mental health experts claim.
>
> A study by the Hunter Child and Youth Mental Health team found that 25 children as young as four, most with ADHD, were being medicated on psychotropic drugs.
>
> Evidence from mental health agencies suggests 65% of children aged 5-18 reported for disruptive behaviour in the Hunter Region were medicated last year.
>
> About 25% of children under five who reported to agencies were medicated.
>
> The figures were revealed as mental health experts expressed

concern about the psychotropic drugs in toddlers, some as young as two, across the State.

Figures from NSW Health show that in NSW alone at least 6,000 children younger than six have been prescribed stimulants over the past decade."

Do we need drugs for kids so-called psyche disorders?

Depression, anxiety, compulsion and behaviour cured naturally

In a personal communication an experienced and caring psychiatrist wrote:

> "The most suicidal patients I ever treated were on Prozac – and they recovered only after getting off Prozac. Many years later I learned of a study where 20% of normal persons became extremely depressed and saw absolutely no reason to live, just 2 or 3 days after taking Prozac. I don't have the data, and so this is hearsay, but I also heard that in the original clinical trials 15% became very suicidal.
>
> Reportedly, Effexor was less effective than a placebo in the original clinical trials. Now the studies have been 'improved' until it is nearly twice as effective as a placebo – using the same drug.
>
> Billions are spent devising ways to alter criteria until the outcome is what they want, and a double-blind, placebo controlled study can be pointed in any direction desired. I no longer trust any of these studies. I see nothing but intentional deception.
>
> Oxycontin was shown on a chart to have a very flat curve. Microscopic print identified the graph as a log rhythmic scale, which can only have a flat curve. Someone complained to the manufacturer that the only purpose for that was deception. The next time they printed the chart they removed the words log rhythmic.
>
> I am very pleased to see the outcome data on 9,000 mental health patients where only 5 recovered after one year. As far as I am concerned, this is evidence that drug treatment is not effective with mental illness."

In January 2002, the *Journal of Pharmopsychiatry* published a paper from the famous Max Planck Institute in Munich. The Institute had been studying the now well known connection between essential fatty acid deficiency, depression,[59] suicide, impulsivity and aggression. Several institutions for young offenders have made similar discoveries in dietary supplement trials of their inmates.

In one recent double-blind study in the UK, 231 young adult prisoners were randomly chosen to either receive a placebo (inactive substance), or a vitamin and mineral supplement together with omega-3 fatty acids. The vitamin and mineral supplement also contained trace elements such as selenium, chromium and manganese. All the nutrients in the supplement were included at levels of more or less the Recommended Daily Dietary Allowance (RDA).

At the start of the trial, the young participants were given psychological tests to measure aggression and their usual dietary intake was determined. The disciplinary offence records of each prisoner before and during the trial were compared.

Promising results

The results of this British study showed that young offenders who received the vitamin and mineral supplement, committed 35% fewer disciplinary offences than those who received the placebo. The most significant improvement was shown in antisocial behaviour which included serious offences such as physical violence.

As it happened

The following testimonies come from an American organization called Safe Harbour, founded by a man who lost his father to 'heroic' psychiatric intervention (electro-convulsive 'therapy'). It is a resource for both professionals and clients who do not wish to go the drug route. I am a member of this group's associated professionals who work with mental health and brain problems. Safe Harbour has an international listing of practitioners and organisations like themselves, which you can find on the internet at www.alternativementalhealth.com

Childhood Panic Disorder

Mother's story of her daughter

I noticed during my daughter Jennifer's early years that any medication labelled 'may cause drowsiness' had the opposite effect. She wasn't hyperactive in the normal sense, but her mind worked overtime. She was reading fluently at four. She had separation anxiety, but attended school from kindergarten through third grade.

Jennifer enjoyed school and was popular with her teachers and the other students. Her annual test scores amazed us all. Then she began having allergies, continual sinusitis and eventually asthma during this time. I consulted an allergist who tested her (skin prick test) for allergies. She came up positive for animals, weeds, trees, grass, mold, dust, etc ... but no food allergies were present. I created kind of a 'clean-room' environment in Jennifer's room, removing the carpet, putting high-efficiency filters (hep A) throughout the house, etc ... and she improved. She still used antihistimines, asthma inhalers and even steroids a few times when the irritation completely closed her nasal passages.

During her third grade year Jennifer began to cry in the morning about going to school. This was accompanied by nausea. We thought she wasn't connecting with her teacher, and might be distressed from boredom due to her advanced abilities. I started home-school, planning to re-enroll her the following year.

Once I began home-schooling Jennifer, I realized how advanced she was. I considered school programs created for bright students, but her separation anxiety and environmental sensitivities kept her home.

When Jennifer was ten, she suddenly became extremely nauseated. It seemed in the beginning to be a virus but it came to stay. Gastro doctor #1 ordered an upper GI, which was inconclusive but traumatic for a ten-year old. Gastro doctor #2 hospitalized her for dehydration. He scheduled Jennifer for a scope test to look into her stomach. He gave her Demerol for the test. It didn't work. He scoped her anyway. Her anxiety became worse. She stayed in the hospital for ten days receiving IV nutrition and medications for gastritis and nausea. When her usable veins were depleted, the doctor wanted to put an IV port in her chest. We refused, and since we saw no improvement, we brought her home.

We then found the Children's Motility Centre at the Children's Hospital, which consisted of a gastroenterologist and a psychologist.

They saw Jennifer and admitted her to Children's Hospital as a nutritional emergency. They prescribed valium. She began to eat. They diagnosed Panic Disorder and prescribed Paxil. They tried several drugs for sleep and found Doxepin made her drowsy. They released Jennifer, suggesting perhaps I should consider a psychiatric hospital for her.

A few days later I found The Panic Disorders Institute. The doctor saw Jennifer immediately, took her off the Paxil and started her on Xanax and Carafate for her stomach. He explained that the sinusitis/asthma was probably caused by refluxing bile, the cause of her gastro-discomfort. Jennifer improved almost immediately and over the next year became functional again.

I began reading about Panic Disorder on the internet and found someone with symptoms identical to what my daughter described. He found he reacted to grain and dairy proteins in a negative way. I took Jennifer off gluten and yeast fifteen months ago.

At the beginning of the dietary change, Jennifer was taking 3mg of Xanax a day, Doxepin at night to sleep and Carafate for her digestion. She is now medication free. She hasn't had a panic attack since I changed her diet.

Jennifer is thirteen now and attends school part time. Her doctor put her on chelated calcium/magnesium, Taurine, Coenzyme Q10 and a multi vitamin. She is happy, socially active, and full of fun, praise God.

She had been in three hospitals, been evaluated by eight doctors, and no one ever suggested diet might be a factor.

Recovery from childhood 'bipolar disorder'

I am the mother of an 11-year-old boy, Lucas, who since birth has shown some symptoms of mental illness. Lucas was always an incredibly active baby who never seemed to need much sleep and literally ran from place to place.

At five years of age, Lucas entered kindergarten – it was somewhat of a disaster. He began having stomach-aches and temper tantrums every morning before going to school. When he entered first grade things got worse. He began wetting himself at school periodically, and had stomach-aches daily that would last until about 4pm when his after-school temper tantrum was played out. Homework was a nightmare beyond belief, the screaming and tears and tantrums were unbelievable.

By third grade Lucas' impulsive behaviors were relentless and his abilities in school were intermittent. He began having sleep-walking episodes and daytime visual/audio hallucinations periodically. I wrongly assumed it was simply stress. His tantrums at home were awesome to behold. The look in his eyes, on his face during these times was animal-like in the extreme, and I couldn't seem to talk with him at the same level after the third grade. The hallucinations and mood swings became more pronounced, to the point where I was becoming very worried about his emotional stability.

In the spring of 2000, he became very depressed and vacillated between a mania/rage so pronounced that he was shoving, hitting, and threatening me; and a depression so severe that I was terrified he would commit suicide. I sought professional help for him. I began to get grey hair that summer, watching Lucas go from insane giggles (as he told me how he was going to kill and dismember me and all his friends) to a state where he couldn't quit laughing and crying at the same time.

It took about 6 weeks for the psychologist I was taking Lucas to see twice a week, to determine that he was bipolar, with attachment issues and obsessive compulsive tendencies with symptoms of attention deficit as well as hyperactivity disorder. I understood that I was expected to administer psychiatric drugs to Lucas (about to turn 11 years old) that had for the most part never been approved for children and that had life threatening side effects, with no experimental evidence indicating that they actually improved the condition in children.

So I began researching alternative medications, and I joined several services for parents of bipolar children. It soon became obvious that almost all of the kids on pharmaceutical drugs ended up in residential care facilities periodically, and the quality of their lives was abysmal. So I decided there had to be a better way – and there was.

The first step was to deal with the depression; we experimented with several different fish oil gel caps as my research indicated that different EPA/DHA ratios were appropriate for different people, and targeted different symptoms. I also began giving him a high quality multivitamin and L-taurine (an amino acid that helps regulate mood) and had found that a couple of herbs truly eliminated the daytime hallucinations, which eliminated most of Lucas's anxiety issues. The restless leg syndrome and sleep walking was effectively dealt with using mineral supplements, particularly magnesium.

I had been reading about the True Hope (TH) supplement, and we decided to try it even though he was relatively stable on the regimen I had set up for him.

Lucas had been eating nutritionally dense foods for a few years, with virtually no dyes or preservatives, as we determined long ago that they affected his health in a negative way. He had also been taking high quality multivitamins and nutritional supplements since the bipolar diagnosis, and sleeping 9 hours a night, but he just didn't seem like the happy-go-lucky kid he had been two years before. Nor did he seem very energetic while taking the pharmaceutical drugs. I hoped the TH supplement would change this, but it did not work for Lucas.

In February, we slowly began lowering the TH supplement and bringing up the quantities of the regimen I had developed through experimentation. The difference in Lucas's life was phenomenal. Suddenly he could sit and read a book again, he could think before speaking or acting on an impulse at a much higher level than ever before.

Lucas has been rock stable since February (six months ago) and his quality of life has never been better. I know this level of responsibility is very difficult to accept. Many a night I would lie awake asking myself what in the world made me think I was capable of handling this without medical professionals? I mean, just who did I think I was? The answer is finally clear, I am Lucas's mother, no more no less, and I have faith that Lucas will have a wonderful childhood with all the same trials and tribulations, all the same opportunities and choices that we want for all children.

ODD and ADD clear on GF–CF Diet

My youngest son, age 17, has suffered with ADD symptoms for many years with the usual problems - obnoxious behaviour that annoyed teachers, family and peers, under achievement and resorting to illicit drugs for comfort.

I found I had celiac disease, a sensitivity to gluten, a protein substance found in wheat and other grains. When I suggested to my older son, who was experiencing severe mental problems, that he stop eating gluten, he noticed an immediate improvement. He got even better after removing milk from his diet.

After seeing the success of his elder brother on the gluten-free diet, my youngest voluntarily began the gluten-free, milk-free diet. After six weeks, he noted how calm he'd become and was enjoying being included in more social activities. He's strictly adhered to the diet for almost 18 months now and his ADD symptoms are well controlled. He's now a senior in high school, succeeding academically, popular with his peers and teachers and happy at home.

Recovery from childhood behaviour problems

My son was diagnosed with 10 different food allergies as an infant. His diet required professional supervision to ensure he ate sufficient fats and vitamins to grow well. As he became a pre-schooler, he did outgrown nine of those allergies, but he maintains a severe dairy allergy at 11 years old, so he continues to be under an allergist's care to monitor this allergy and his mild asthma.

By the time he entered kindergarten, we blamed a lot of his behaviour on his asthma. We noticed he seemed to have a tantrum often before an asthma attack, but the allergist assured us that this was unrelated. Still, I am not sure. By second grade, the school was implying he had ADD, though we really did not believe this. We had him evaluated by two developmental paediatricians, who would commit to nothing other than to tell us he was perhaps borderline hyperactive/ADD. One of them recommended we read a book about hidden food allergies, but our allergist denied that the book had any merit. Still, we read it and learned about the food dye -behaviour connection. Later, the allergist agreed that this connection is real, but it is a chemical reaction rather than an allergic reaction.

At this time, serendipitously, we ran into another family who was reading labels at a party to check for ingredients. We offered to share our chocolate soy milk, if it was a dairy issue. However, we learned that their daughter avoided Red Dye #40. When we asked what would happen to her, her mother hesitated and then shared that her daughter's behaviour would dramatically change. She would throw a loud, aggressive tantrum after eating Red Dye #40. I had heard of this before, and had really resisted having to go organic, since our diet had already been so dramatically altered due to the food allergies.

However, my husband and I could not deny that this was something we should check into after we gave him a red candy for a treat at an event serving only dairy and junk foods, and within fifteen minutes he was swearing, kicking, and just downright rude. We experimented; completely avoiding it and then letting him have it. It was like turning a light switch on and off, 'good behaviour' and then 'bad behaviour'. These tantrums were such that we would put him in his bedroom and he would just kick the door and swear and then later he would just say, "Can I come out? I feel better."

Car trips were always a horrible nightmare for us, with his continual tantrums after about an hour. Then, we realized that we always served him juice boxes in the car, with artificial Red Dye #40 in it! Now, we can go for four or five hour trips without more than the "normal" restlessness. It is incredible. When I think back to how many tears I cried out of frustration and how much I would have to fight the urge to leave him on the side of the road....well, that is why I am writing this!

He is now in fifth grade, and voluntarily avoids artificial red foods. He just shrugs and tells people, "You don't know wanna know what will happen to me if I eat that! Really, I will just go nuts." But the sad part is, there's got to be lots of kids out there that do "go nuts" and they may not be as fortunate as our son to have parents that figured this out. They may be suffering and getting into trouble with their families, schools, and even the police. When you realize that it is lower income, less educated families that eat more of the junk food it compounds the issue.

Years ago, I worked with emotionally disturbed children, and I know we fed them artificial colours, and I remember seeing this kind of behaviour at that group home. How many of them could have been managed at home with healthier diets? I think it is outrageous.

Recovery from depression

I was diagnosed with depression when I was 18 and spent 3 weeks in a mental hospital. I was on psychiatric drugs for 10 months after that. The drugs made me feel lethargic, impatient and irritable. They also clouded my thinking and made it impossible for me to sleep deeply. Even so, I tried psychiatric drugs a couple more times after that because I was so convinced by the 'experts' (psychiatrists, psychotherapists and their books) that I had some fundamental brain chemistry problem and their drugs were my only hope. I didn't have any idea what else to do.

Years later, I was diagnosed with Chronic Fatigue Syndrome (I have the cytomegalovirus) as well as debilitating food allergies to foods I've eaten every day of my life! This was the true cause of my depression. I happened upon *The cure for all diseases* by Dr. Hulda Clark. I killed parasites and viruses according to her instructions and cleaned my kidneys and liver. With each liver cleanse, my vitality, strength and metabolism returned. My food allergies disappeared. Life becomes brighter. I became motivated and optimistic. I began to feel like the old me from a long, long time ago.

I can express how grateful am I to have truly solved my health problems. I am able to live once again. I have passed this book on to many of my friends.

Candida-induced anxiety

I was terribly afraid of what was happening to me, as I was unaware that there was any physiological or medical condition causing these symptoms. I sought a doctor's help; then two, then three. In all three instances, I was quickly examined and upon hearing my laundry list of symptoms, I was offered psychiatric meds as the solution to what they considered ailed me – my mind. I declined the drugs in each instance, convinced that the physicians didn't have a clue what was really happening with me.

After 9 months of this torture and fear, it was recommended to me to go to a chiropractor who applied nutrition testing to his patients. He determined, through this testing, that my body was full of yeast and the high-sugar fruits I was eating were feeding the yeast, causing them to multiply and affect me on a continuing and unrelenting basis.

The chiropractor put me on a diet that prohibited yeast or fermented products, sugar, cheese, and dairy. It took 3 weeks of religiously following the diet to kill the yeast, but I did. Actually, within a week, I was feeling much better. I've not experienced any more of those symptoms since.

I owe that chiropractor a lot for correctly assessing my situation and for not assuming that it was all in my head and that a prescription of Prozac would make it all go away!

PART THREE

Nutritional program and recipes

CHAPTER SEVENTEEN

The ADD/HD nutritional program

Some protein foods for ASD children under treatment

Casein and Gluten-Free

Eggs (free-range)
Fish (must have fins and scales in the wild – not smooth-skin fish) such as salmon, sardines, mackerel, cod, barramundi, hoki, herring, bream and tuna
Vegetarian Protein
Sanitarium 'BBQ soy sausages' (kid's favourite!)
Nutolene
Nutal burgers, chick peas (complete protein) or falafel
Tofu (slice and marinate with soy sauce)
Tempeh
Soy beans (complete protein)
Lentils and all beans (these need another protein to complete, such as peanuts/butter, tahini, sunflower, or add egg, or nuts such as pecan, walnut, almonds, brazil)
Soy yoghurt or soy ice-cream
Hommus
Avocado dip (with fetta cheese)
Nut spreads
Tahini
Soy cheese
Peanut butter (freshly roasted and ground form your local health food shop, contains no chemicals, or Sanitarium natural peanut butter)
Nut spreads such as almond butter, cashew – but NOT 'Nutella'!
Do NOT use margarine – use ButterSoft (Mainland brand) for the whole family

Become a label reader. Watch for gluten; casein; GM (genetically modified); MSG (monosodium glutamate, also declared as flavour enhancer 621); and other chemicals including colouring and flavouring. Most of these can be found in any chemical guide booklet – take one shopping, like a golfer asks his caddy for advice!

Foods to avoid on a candida diet

Try to eat none of these foods for one month and then see your health practitioner for a re-assessment. Remember, the foods above the line specifically feed *Candida albicans*.

- All sugars and fruits, including: raw or refined sugar, honey or foods containing sugars (commercial juices, cordials, most breakfast cereals, etc); dried fruits of all kinds (raisins, figs, prunes, etc.). Read the labels on all foods!
- Malted foods, such as sweets with malt, Horlicks, malted breakfast cereals, malted milkshakes, malted chocolat drinks, etc.

Foods to which a person with candidiasis will be allergic, although they do not actually feed *Candida albicans*.

- Fermented beverages, especially beer and wine; whisky, brandy, gin, rum, vodka, cider, etc.
- Ferments/moulds, such as soya sauce, Vegemite, Promite, Marmite, miso, mushrooms. Other foods with mould include: cantaloupes, melons, oranges, dried fruits of all kinds (raisins, figs, prunes, etc.), pickled and smoked foods (especially frankfurters), corned beef, devon, etc.
  Also, stale or stored foods – packet foods left open must be eaten fresh. Canned juices, especially tomato and apple.
- Raised (yeasted) breads and doughs: breads, buns, rolls, pastries, biscuits (except those allowed under 'Foods to eat'); cakes, cake mixes, etc.
- Vinegars; salad dressing (use lemon juice instead); mayonnaise; pickles; olives; most sauces of all kinds including chilli, pickled beets, relishes, etc.
- Dairy products: everything from the cow – milk, cream, matured cheese, sour cream, etc. Noted exceptions are yoghurt, buttermilk and 'soft butter'.
- Brewer's yeast and all other types of yeast – including torula, and vitamins containing yeast.
- Stored nuts, especially peanuts, but freshly shelled nuts are all right. No peanut butter.
- Coffee, tea and cola drinks
- Antibiotics

Foods to eat

These foods either kill or inhibit candida include: raw garlic, onion, kale, turnips, cabbage, horseradish and broccoli.

Foods in this list marked * are protein foods.

- All vegetables (especially globe artichokes which help repair damaged intestinal walls);
- Young lean meat (if meat eater)*;
- Free-range chicken*;
- Fish*;
- Free range eggs*;
- Legumes of all kinds (soya beans, lentils, lima, barlotti, navy beans)*;
- Brown rice and other wholegrain unyeasted foods, for example: Ryvita, Vitaweet, rice cakes, waffles made from whole grains and buckwheat (see Recipe section), matzo (Jewish) unleavened bread, millet biscuits and wholegrain freshly ground porridge, etc.;
- Complex carbohydrates (of which the above grain foods mostly consist), including full-grain rye bread, yeast-free Demeter bread, potatoes, pasta (especially wholegrain spaghetti, etc.);
- Goat's milk products, sugar-free soya milk, plain yoghurt (Attiki or Jalna biodynamic if possible)*
- Herb teas, dandelion coffee, etc.;
- Nuts and seeds (such as sunflower or sesame) and tahini paste.*;
- Homemade salad dressings (with lemon and garlic, etc.);
- Grapefruit and lemon allowed;
- Packaged foods should be opened when you are ready to eat and left-overs stored in an airtight container;
- Tinned fish – eat freshly opened*;
- Homemade soups/broths – eat when fresh;
- Popcorn;
- Twice baked bread ('Zwiebak').

Note: In fact, you can eat almost any food not found in the 'Foods to avoid' list. And must make sure you eat enough! If you cut out foods you must replace them adequately.

Note on program

Remember that this program is not 'for the term of your natural life', although it is nutritionally very sound and many well informed vegetarians live long lives on it – without the chicken and sometimes without the fish.

For at least one month, this program should be adhered to strictly. Severe and chronic sufferers will have to remain on the program longer.

Withdrawals

If you have been a consistent coffee or tea drinker you may experience headaches and/or nausea for a day or so. Try to dilute your particular drink, gradually diluting further and adding dandelion coffee or similar to your coffee, and peppermint tea or similar to your tea.

Possible allergens among the above

Some patients will have trouble with foods that are normally acceptable to other allergy victims. This is because of biological individuality. Below is a short list of some of the most common allergens:

- deadly nightshade family (such as tomatoes, potatoes, capsicums);
- salicylate family (all fruits except skinned pears), plus tomatoes, capsicum, zucchini, cucumber, gherkin, chilli, baked beans, almonds, honey, most herbs and spices, carrots, oranges, bananas and tinned fruit.

'Sick buildings'

Research studies over a period of several decades show that people who live or work in closed spaces and in environments containing more positive airborne ions than negative ions (such as air-conditioned buildings), may develop a variety of symptoms. Typical manifestations include fatigue, headache, drowsiness, irritability, nasal discharge, burning eyes and coughing. These and other symptoms commonly found in individuals with yeast-connected health disorders may be helped by a negative ion generator.

Easy to follow daily eating program

On arising

Two to three glasses of spring water, filtered or rain water, in which you have soaked some slices of lemon – including skin – overnight. Add hot water to make warm.

Breakfast

Make breakfast your main meal rather than at dinner time. This meal reversal is most important for all digestive tract problems.

- Choose recipe from Salads;
- One from Protein Dishes or Fish. Those who retain meat in the diet can also have it at this meal, but should certainly have it no later than lunchtime;
- One from Vegetables;
- One from Staple Dishes.

Those who work and can't manage a meal like this should at least have protein and some raw vegetables before leaving for work, or take some sandwiches for on the way. This is important.

Lunch

- Choose from Salads;
- One from Grains and Desserts.

Evening meal

Make this a light meal.

- Choose one from Soups;
- One from Salads;
- Crispbread such as Kavli, Ryvita, matzo, sesame crackers or Scottish Oatcakes (see Recipe section).

Comments on the daily eating program

The suggested menu has been scientifically compiled. The reasons for making breakfast your main meal are:

- The peak performance of your stomach is between 7–9am (between 5–7pm is the peak performance of the kidneys).
- The body is most active after breakfast, until about 3pm, when it begins to slow down. This includes the digestive tract as well as every other system. Therefore, the transit time of the food you have eaten at breakfast is likely to be shorter, which is important, particularly with putrefactive foods such as meat and other proteins, and cooked food.
- Your blood sugar level is below normal on arising. If you do not eat

any breakfast it will stay at this lowered rate, and you will be working on your reserves.

If you eat the usual sweet breakfast, high in simple carbohydrate, or even fruit, your blood sugar level will rise quickly, but will then drop rapidly and be below normal again. With this sudden drop in blood sugar you will also feel a lack of energy, tiredness and a desire for something sweet by morning teatime. If you have protein for breakfast, combined with raw or slightly cooked vegetables, you will not have this problem. We have had many patients suffering from hypoglycaemia (low blood sugar) in our clinic. They have done very well on this breakfast.

It is easier for you to resist eating sweets and fruits if you eat a *good protein breakfast and nothing sweet.*

- Because your body is active earlier in the day, having your main meal for breakfast fits in very well with a weight control program. The food metabolises better and you will be less inclined to 'pick' in-between meals, since a normal blood sugar level will prevent you from feeling hungry.

Reasons for making your evening meal light are:

- Your body is tired after a day's work – this includes your stomach. It is not wise to eat large heavy meals when tired. Very often the food just sits in the stomach all night, often causing colic, especially in children.
- The body has slowed down, as has the digestive system. It will therefore take much longer to digest a meal – especially a heavy meal such as meat and cooked vegetables.
- When going to bed with a full stomach and food only half digested, you will have a restless, poor quality sleep. This affects your nervous system adversely. To have a good quality sleep the stomach should not be full but at rest, the same as the rest of the body.
- A large, heavy meal with no activity or very little after it, tends to cause weight problems. It will also cause constipation, the root of many chronic diseases.
- When you have eaten a large, heavy meal at night, you will feel lethargic on waking and you will not be ready for a proper breakfast. It is like a hangover.

To switch over to this menu it is wise to start making the evening meal lighter first, and then gradually increasing your breakfast. It takes time to change the routine, especially if you are the cook. Plan your breakfast the day before. Make casseroles or patty mixes, which can be stored in the fridge or freezer, ready to cook in the morning. Tossed salads can be kept in airtight containers or similar.

Once you have planned everything this way you will feel the freedom of not having to rush home to cook a meal when you are out somewhere; and you won't tire yourself out cooking at the end of the day, then eating, and then having to do the dishes. But, most important of all, the health of the family will improve.

Gastro-intestinal peak times in bio-chronology

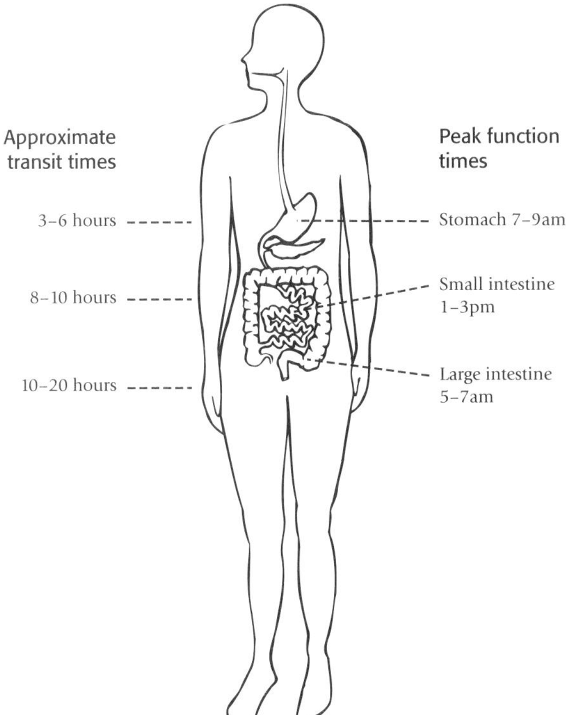

American psycho-biologist Professor Kurt Richter discovered the biorhythm timing of various organs in the late 1920s. Oriental medicine had by that time already been using this knowledge for thousands of years!

CHAPTER EIGHTEEN

Seven-day step-by-step menu plan

Using the seven-day menu is a good way to get started on the program. It is designed to commence on Sunday, so that you have time to shop and make preparations on Saturday, rather than trying to start the program in the middle of the week, which for most people is a more hectic time. The program can be modified to suit individual needs and tastes.

Saturday, before starting menu plan

Prepare for Sunday:

soak mung beans overnight
coleslaw (put in airtight container in fridge)
Scottish oatcakes, if desired

Buy necessary vegetables for Sunday and Monday

Where you have little time for preparations during the weekdays, it is all right to make a number of protein dishes during the weekend to keep in the freezer. Take the casserole of your choice for the next morning out of the freezer the evening before.

Sunday

On arising 2–3 glasses warm lemon drink.

Breakfast (main meal)

fried rice (or barley if allergic to rice)
mung beans
coleslaw
sugar snap peas

Lunch

cornmeal pancakes, waffles or pikelets
salmon toss

Evening meal (light)

pumpkin soup
gluten-free crispbread
salad with cold pressed olive oil dressing

Prepare for Monday

easy bread *gluten-free*
sesame crackers
barlotti bean loaf

Monday

On arising 2–3 glasses warm lemon drink.

Breakfast

spiced potatoes
barlotti bean loaf
spinach salad
brussels sprouts

Lunch

easy bread *gluten-free*
pumpernickel (very dark, thinly sliced rye bread) *not gluten-free*
waldorf salad

Evening meal

celery soup
sesame crackers or rice cakes
salad with cold pressed olive oil dressing

Prepare for Tuesday

buy necessary vegetables
beetroot salad

Tuesday

On arising 2–3 glasses warm lemon drink.

Breakfast

chick peas and spinach pasta
marinated grilled fish
peas and carrots
beetroot salad

Lunch

some hors d'oeuvres bites
sour dough bread *gluten-free*
matzos
almonds

Dinner

red lentil soup
variety of crispbread
salad with cold pressed olive oil dressing

Prepare for Wednesday

buy necessary vegetables
lentil patty mixture
green bean salad

Wednesday

On arising 2–3 glasses warm lemon drink.

Breakfast

buckwheat roast
lentil patties
broccoli
green bean salad (add yoghurt)

Lunch

radish salad
milk porridge or scones (*gluten-free,* see recipes)
pepitas

Dinner

beetroot soup
crisp bread (*gluten-free*) such as rice snaps
small butternut salad

Prepare for Thursday

buy necessary vegetables
chick pea casserole
red cabbage salad
easy bread *gluten-free*

Thursday

On arising 2–3 glasses warm lemon drink.

Breakfast

potato pancakes
chick pea casserole
cauliflower
red cabbage salad

Lunch

carrot salad
easy bread *gluten-free*
pecan nuts

Dinner

vegetable soup
corn-on-cob
salad with cold pressed olive oil dressing

Prepare for Friday

buy necessary vegetables
beetroot salad
cornbread cakes
soak cannelini beans overnight

Friday

On arising 2–3 glasses warm lemon drink.

Breakfast

savoury millet
oven-baked ocean bream
beetroot salad
sugar snap peas and baby carrots

Lunch

hors d'oeuvres bites
corn bread cakes
pumpernickel

Dinner

cannelini bean soup
crisp bread (gluten-free) such as rice snaps
salad with cold pressed olive oil dressing

Prepare for Saturday

buy necessary vegetables
nut galantine
pumpkin pie
rice salad
asparagus salad (cover with food wrap)
sesame crackers

Saturday

On arising 2–3 glasses warm lemon drink.

Breakfast

potato casserole
asparagus salad
nut galantine
red cabbage

Lunch

rice salad
pumpkin pie or carob pudding

Dinner

choko soup or spinach soup
sesame crackers
parsnip salad (small)

Prepare for Sunday

buy necessary vegetables for Sunday and Monday
prepare planned casseroles and salads and also baking

Product information

Foods

Most products should be available from your supermarket.

Agar agar

A natural jelly derived from the sea.

Artificial sweetener/sugar substitute

Use sparingly and try to obtain the most natural powder, nothing containing sorbitol, cyclamate or aspartame. If you need a sweetener, try Stevia in liquid or powder form. Stevia is a natural, plant-derived product. It is 30 times sweeter than sugar, extremely low in calories and will not feed candida. Available from health food shops.

Barley flour

Use for thickening soups and sauces. Available from health food shops.

Basil, fresh

Best grown with tomatoes to keep off bugs.

Basil, dried

Has a flavour similar to black pepper, but not the harmful effect that pepper has on the stomach lining.

Bay leaf

Apart from flavouring soups and stews, it stops flatulence.

Cloves

Same effect as bay leaf.

Cold pressed oil (preferably olive oil)

This oil is extracted without the use of heat, or chemicals. Some are very rich in linoleic acid, a necessary substance for digestion. Most cooking oils produce oxidants when heated. Oxidants are precursors to many diseases including cancer. Cold pressed olive oil is an exception – it is a mono-saturated, CIS fatty acid and recommended. Use of garlic or onion in cooking oil reduces oxidant risk.

Cottage cheese
This is easier to digest than milk or hard cheeses. All soured milk products are easier to digest because of bacterial action. However, some allergy patients cannot tolerate even these dairy foods because of their lactose content.

Egg replacer (Orgran)
Use 1 heaped teaspoon mixed with 2 tablespoons water to replace *one* egg. Available from health food shops.

Garlic
Garlic is an important flavouring agent. When cooking, always finish frying before adding garlic, to avoid it taking on a bitter taste.

Goat's milk
Easier to digest than cow's milk and much healthier, but not tolerated by some allergy patients. Use fresh for better taste.

Low-allergy baking powder
It does not have the harmful ingredients you find in other baking powders and agrees with most people suffering from allergies. Available from health food shops.

Pepitas
Green pumpkin seeds with a nutty taste. Available from health food shops.

Rice flour
Use for thickening soups and sauces as well as for baking. Available from health food shops.

Soft butter (Mainland)
Pure-cream butter, slightly whipped to make it spreadable direct from the fridge.

Sour cream
See 'Cottage cheese'.

Soya mayonnaise (Norganic)
An organic, dairy-free mayonnaise.

Soya milk
A non-dairy substitute for milk.

Stock powder (Massel)
Available in 3 flavours – vegetable, beef, chicken – but contains neither animal ingredients, nor MSG. Can also be used as seasoning.

Tahini
Sesame paste can be used as bread spread or in casserole dishes.

Tofu
Soya bean curd. Cut into cubes and marinade in soy sauce overnight. Fry with a little soft butter until brown.

Turmeric
A yellow powdered herb with a curry-like flavour. If you are not allergic to this it is a good substitute for curry. To make it hot you'll need to add cayenne pepper as well.

TVP
Textured Vegetable Protein, made from soya beans. Some added ingredients could be allergenic.

Water purifier
Drinking treated town water from your tap will hinder your progress. Chlorine (added to all town water) has a very destructive effect on your intestinal flora. A water purifier is a good health investment.

Wheatgerm
This part of the wheat contains the Vitamin E. If you are allergic to wheatgerm, rolled millet can be substituted for it.

Yoghurt
Easily make your won with Natren's Yogurt Starter, a bottle which will make up to 10 litres of delicious Bulgarian-style yoghurt. Alternatively, buy a good continental quality such as Attiki or Jalna. Yoghurt is a very healthy food for those who can tolerate it.

Supplements

These are mostly only available from health food shops.

Colloidal minerals
A multi-mineral supplement that helps with allergies. It contains a mineral balance very similar to that found in the human body plus essential trace elements often missing from our western diet. These minerals and trace elements are in a colloidal form, which means they have been processed by plants and therefore easlily absorbed by your body. They are pollution-free, having been formed prehistorically, and found by researchers to chelate or clean-out toxic metals from patients. In Australia colloidal minerals supplements have been successfully used to help overcome chemical toxicity and alleviate serious allergies in people when taken regularly.

Garlic
Garlic is a natural anti-biotic substance. The best way to take garlic as a nutritional supplement is in aged liquid form – it retains all of garlic's beneficial properties, but has none of the harsh substances.

Spirulina
This is a single-cell micro algae that grows in warm, fresh water. It is the single most nutritious food source known to man and richest of any whole food in the following organic immune-boosting nutrients:

- *Beta-carotene*
  A powerful anti-oxidant that protects all other anti-oxidants (substances that prevent disease processes and ageing). *The Journal of Nutrition*, July 1989, published a study showing organic beta-carotene to have a 10-fold higher assimilation and biological activity than synthetic beta-carotene.
  Currently, the average intake of beta-carotene is only 4mg daily In the US, but the National Cancer Institute is recommending 6mg as the minimum daily requirement. This is because beta-carotene has been shown to protect against cancer of the lung and other cancers in very large population studies.
  New studies show that beta-carotene can restore communication pathways between cell walls that transmit normal growth signals. It can thus normalise abnormal cell growth.
  Hawaiian Pacifica Spirulina is the only organic spirulina brand used by most practitioners. It supplies you with about 12mg of beta-carotene in an average daily dose.
- *Iron*
  Population studies in the Western world invariably show that very high percentages of women suffer from mild to severe iron deficiency. Ten percent of the Spirulina content is iron, the highest source by far of any food. Moreover, it is organic iron, 94 percent assimilable and will not cause constipation – unlike many iron supplements.
- *B12*
  Spirulina contains more than four times the quantity found in beef liver.
- *Calcium*
  Twice as much as in sesame seeds or parsley – the closest rivals.
- *Amino Acids*
  Twice as rich as soya beans in protein, Spirulina is 60 percent high-quality protein.

Natradophilus, BifidoFactor and LifeStart

Three friendly bacteria supplements from Natren – no other product supplies as many organisms per gram guaranteed. These living foods possess unique abilities to enhance natural immunity, restore the level of friendly bacteria in the small and large intestine and supply B vitamins. LifeStart is specifically developed for children ages 0–7.

Probioplex

An antibody concentrate made from whey. It eliminates over 40 pathogenic intestinal organisms responsible for diarrhoea and mucosal inflammations.

Probioplex helps the friendly bacteria, like acidophilus and bifidus, to adhere to your bowel walls and colonise.

Probioplex also enhances the activity of these friendly bacteria in eliminating *Candida albicans* and other enemies.

CHAPTER NINETEEN

Recipe suggestions

All recipes can be made gluten-free and/or casein-free, unless otherwise noted. All mammal's milk contains casein.

Soups

Vegetable soup

Variety of vegetables such as carrots, peas, beans, cauliflower, parsley celery leeks, etc.

1 1/4 litres (5 cups) water
1/4 cup cooked brown rice or vermicelli
2 tablespoons cold pressed oil
1/4 teaspoon nutmeg
1/4 teaspoon dried basil
pinch cayenne pepper
2 Massel seasoning cubes

Wash vegetables and cut into small pieces. Sauté in oil for 10 minutes. Add water and rice or vermicelli and simmer for 30 minutes. Add the herbs to taste.

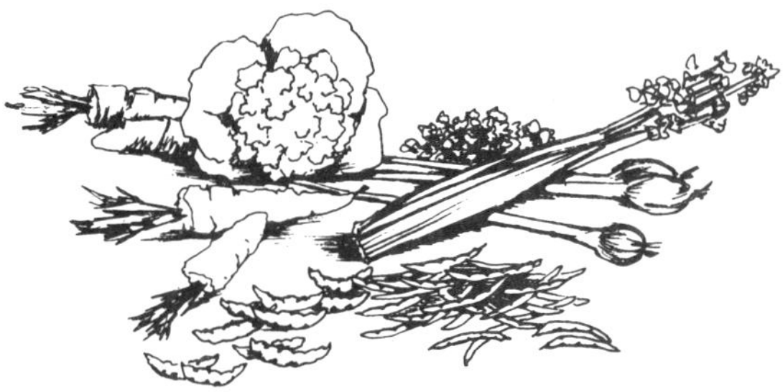

Potato soup

4 potatoes (or sweet potatoes)
3/4 litre (3 cups) water
1 cup goat's milk or soya milk
1 teaspoon cold pressed oil
1 cup chopped leeks
1/4 cup coarsely grated carrot
1/4 cup chopped celery (inc leaves)
2 Massel seasoning cubes
pinch cayenne pepper
1/2 teaspoon nutmeg

Scrub potatoes, cut in pieces, including skin, and cook in water until soft. Put potatoes and remaining cooking liquid through a strainer and add milk. Sauté vegetables in oil with Massel seasoning, cayenne pepper and nutmeg for about 10 minutes and add to the potatoes.

Sweet corn soup

1 onion, finely chopped
1 clove garlic, crushed
1 tablespoon cold pressed oil
2 tablespoons rice flour
1 litre (4 cups) water
1 cup sweet corn, mashed
1 egg yolk, beaten (optional)
2 Massel seasoning cubes
¼ cup chopped parsley
2 tablespoons yoghurt (optional)

Sauté onion and garlic in hot oil until onion is transparent. Add rice flour and gradually stir in half the water. Add egg yolk, corn and Massel seasoning and simmer for 10 minutes. Just before serving add parsley and yoghurt.

Spinach soup

2 cups finely shredded spinach
¾ litre (3 cups) water
1 tablespoon cold pressed olive oil
1 onion, chopped
2 tablespoons rice flour
½ cup goat's milk or soya milk
pinch cayenne pepper
1 teaspoon dried basil
½ teaspoon nutmeg
2 Massel seasoning cubes
rice snaps, for serving

Wash and cook spinach in 1 cup of water for about 5 minutes on low heat. Put through blender, retaining any remaining cooking liquid. Heat oil, sauté onion until transparent, then add flour and remaining water while constantly stirring. Add spinach and other ingredients. Simmer for 10 minutes and serve with rice snaps.

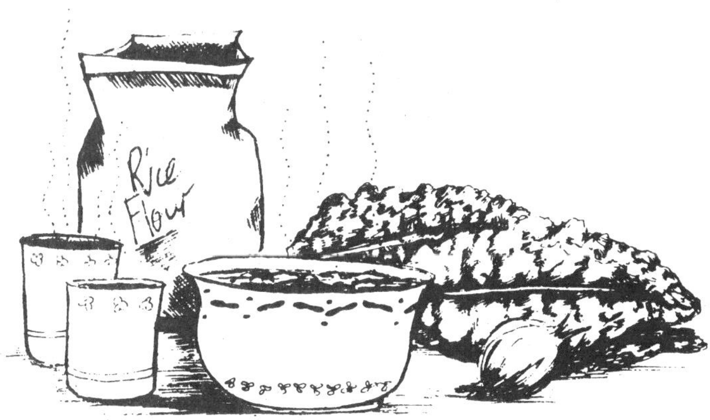

Carrot soup

1 onion
1 tablespoon cold pressed oil
2 tablespoons rice or barley flour
¾ litre (3 cups) water
½ cup cooked mashed carrots
½ cup peas
1 cup of goat's or soya milk
2 Massel seasoning cubes
pinch cayenne pepper
1 teaspoon dried basil
½ teaspoon oregano
¼ cup finely chopped parsley

Chop onion and sauté in hot oil until transparent. Using French whisk, add flour while gradually adding water. Add other ingredients and simmer for 10 minutes. Lastly add parsley.

Celery soup

1 onion
1 cup chopped celery
1 tablespoon cold pressed oil
3 tablespoons rice flour
¾ litre (3 cups) water
½ cup goat's milk or soya milk
2 Massel seasoning cubes
¼ cup chopped celery leaves
2–3 tablespoons of yoghurt

Chop onion and sauté with celery in hot oil until onion transparent. Using a French whisk, add flour and gradually stir in the water. Simmer until celery is soft. Strain if required. Add milk, Massel seasoning and celery leaves. Before serving stir in yoghurt.

Tomato soup

3–4 tomatoes (unsprayed)
1 small bay leaf
2 cloves
¾ litre (3 cups) water
1 onion
1 tablespoon cold pressed oil
2 tablespoons rice or barley flour
1 cup goat's or soya milk
pinch of cayenne pepper
2 tablespoons fresh basil, chopped
2 tablespoons parsley leaves
2 Massel seasoning cubes
2 tablespoons yoghurt

Simmer tomatoes with bay leaf and cloves in some of the water until soft. Put through strainer, retaining any remaining cooking liquid. Chop onion and sauté until transparent. Add flour and then gradually add the remaining water while stirring. Add the milk, cayenne, basil and parsley or celery leaves. Salt to taste. Simmer for a few minutes and add yoghurt before serving.

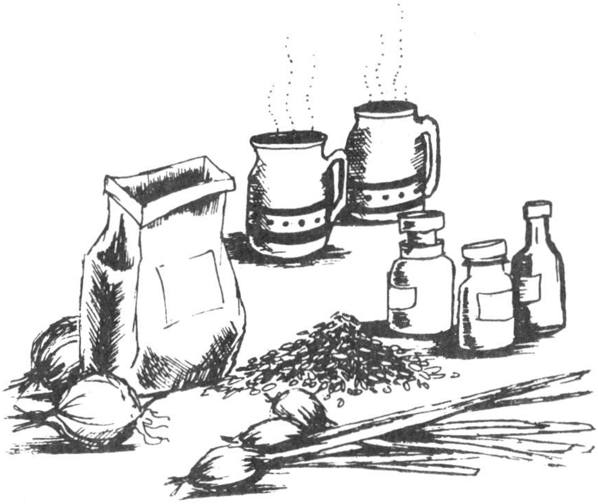

Red lentil soup

½ cup red lentils
1 carrot, coarsely grated
1 litre (4 cups) water
1 bay leaf
1 onion
1 tablespoon of safflower oil
little thyme and turmeric
2 Massel seasoning cubes
squeeze lemon juice

Cook lentils and carrot in the water with the bay leaf for 15 minutes or until soft. Chop onion and sauté in hot oil with herbs for 10 minutes. Add to the lentils along with the rest of water and other ingredients. Simmer for about ½ hour. Serve with seaweed or plain rice snaps.

Kidney bean soup

½ cup kidney or barlotti beans
1 litre (4 cups) water
3 cloves
1 bay leaf
1 large onion
1 leek
1 celery stalk with leaves, chopped
1 tablespoon cold pressed oil
1 teaspoon turmeric
½ teaspoon thyme
½ teaspoon nutmeg
1 teaspoon dried basil
pinch cayenne pepper
1 tablespoon rice or barley flour
2 Massel seasoning cubes

Soak beans in the water for 24 hours with cloves and bay leaf. Cook them until soft, then mash them or use blender. Chop and sauté onion, leeks and celery stalks in hot oil for about 10 minutes. Add to the beans the herbs, spices and rice or barley flour, Massel seasoning, salt and chopped celery leaves. Simmer for 15 minutes.

Cannelini bean soup

½ cup cannelini or haricot beans
1 litre (4 cups) water
1 onion
1 leek
1 tablespoon cold pressed oil
1 tablespoon rice or barley flour
2 Massel seasoning cubes
vegetable salt to taste
½ teaspoon nutmeg
pinch cayenne pepper

Soak beans in water for 24 hours. Bring to boil, and cook for about 1½ hours or until soft. Chop onion and leeks and sauté in hot oil for a few minutes. Add together with barley or rice flour to the beans, add Massel seasoning, salt, nutmeg and cayenne pepper. Simmer till creamy.

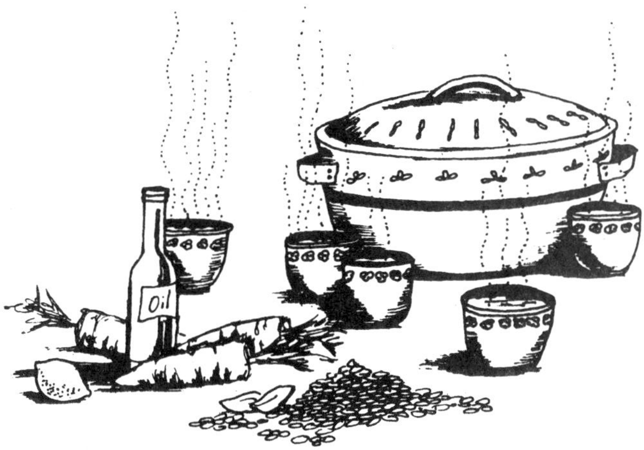

Pumpkin soup

2 cups diced butternut pumpkin (including skin)
¾ litre (3 cups) water
1 cup goat's or soya milk
1 small onion
1 tablespoon cold pressed oil
2 tablespoons rice or barley flour
2 Massel seasoning cubes
1 teaspoon dried basil
½ teaspoon nutmeg
pinch cayenne pepper
parsley, very finely chopped
1 tablespoon yoghurt

Cook pumpkin in the water until soft, then mash. Add rice or barley flour while stirring with French whisk. Sauté onion in hot oil for 10 minutes. Add together with herbs, Massel seasoning and milk. Before serving on each plate add yoghurt.

Asparagus soup

250 g (½ lb) asparagus
¾ litre (3 cups) water
1 tablespoon cold pressed oil
2 tablespoons rice or barley flour
1 egg yolk (optional)
1 cup goat's or soya milk
½ teaspoon nutmeg
2 Massel seasoning cubes
2 tablespoons yoghurt

Wash asparagus, cut off heads, cut stalks into small pieces and soak in half the water until soft. Rub through strainer, retaining any remaining liquid. Heat oil, add the flour and stir with French whisk or wooden spoon while adding the remaining water. Add the asparagus heads, then add other ingredients except the yoghurt. Simmer until asparagus heads are soft. Add yoghurt before serving.

Note: If fresh asparagus is unavailable, use tinned asparagus.

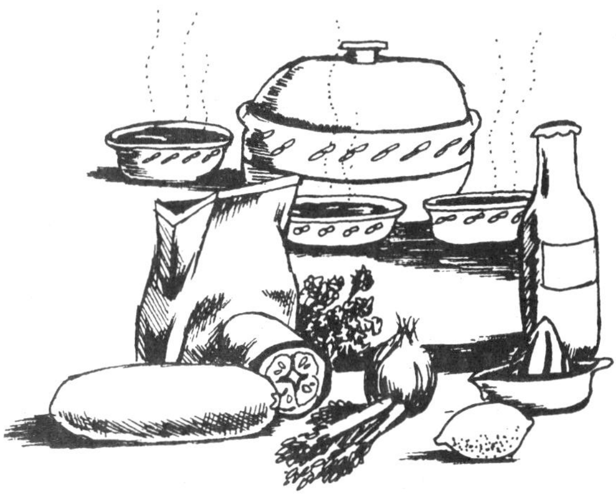

Beetroot soup (borsch)

¾ litre (3 cups) water
1 beetroot, grated
1 carrot, grated
1 large onion, chopped
1 cup chopped celery
1 cup cooked lima or haricot beans
2 Massel seasoning cubes
2 tablespoons chopped parsley
1 tablespoon fresh dill, chopped or 1 teaspoon dried dill tips
1 tablespoon lemon juice
2 tablespoons yoghurt

Bring water to boil with all ingredients except last four. Simmer until soft, then add parsley, dill and lemon juice. Stir in yoghurt just before serving.

Cucumber or choko soup

2 cups chopped cucumber or choko
¾ litre (3 cups) water
1 onion, chopped very finely
1 clove garlic, crushed
1 tablespoon cold-pressed safflower oil
2 tablespoons rice or barley flour
½ cup goat's or soya milk
2 Massel seasoning cubes
1 teaspoon lemon juice
1 tablespoon dill or 2 tablespoons parsley, chopped
2 tablespoons yoghurt

Cook cucumber or choko with some of the water till soft. Blend and strain. Sauté onion and garlic in oil until onion transparent, then, using French whisk, add rice or barley flour and stir in remaining water and milk. Add Massel seasoning and lemon juice. Just before serving stir dill or parsley and yoghurt through.

Summer soup

½ cucumber
1 cup fresh peas
2–3 asparagus
1 spring onion
1 tablespoon cold pressed oil
2 tablespoons rice flour
¾ litre (3 cups) water
2 Massel seasoning cubes
1 cup goat's or soya milk
2 tablespoons chopped fresh basil
2 tablespoons chopped parsley
squeeze of lemon juice

Finely chop vegetables and sauté in oil for 5 minutes. Add flour, then water gradually while stirring and then add Massel seasoning. Simmer until vegetables are soft. Add milk, basil and parsley then lemon juice and simmer for 5 minutes.

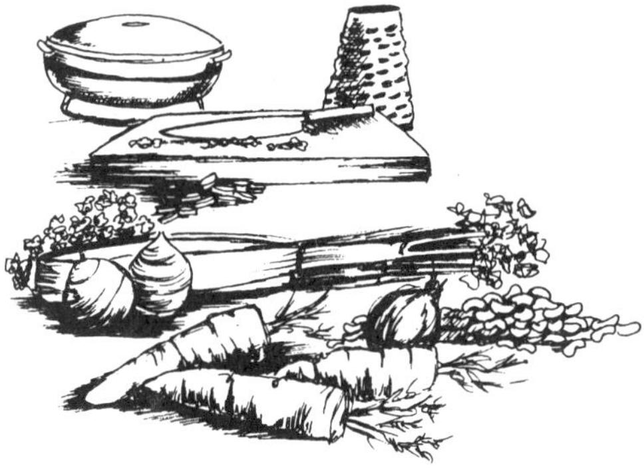

Salads

Hors d'oeuvres platter (bites)

Rub garlic on platter before choosing some of the following:

- 5 cm (2") celery pieces filled with a mixture of cottage cheese and chives.
- 5 cm (2") celery pieces, made into curls by splitting down each side into thin sections, but leaving attached at base, then placing in iced water for about 1 hour.
- Carrots sliced lengthwise to make sticks.
- Radishes cut in slices, roses, quarters or used whole. Leave a few small middle leaves on and slice across bottom to stand up.
- Tomato slices or quarters. Put whole tomatoes in boiling water for a few minutes to be able to remove skin. Then slice or quarter and marinade in a mixture of cold pressed oil, lemon juice, basil and vegetable salt. Arrange on a platter. Top with finely chopped parsley.
- Cucumber slices. Marinade the same way as tomatoes.
- Sardines, slightly smoked or plain.
- Sliced cooked beetroot marinated as tomatoes.
- Olives.
- Cottage cheese balls. Mix cottage cheese with a little yoghurt and grated nuts. Form into small balls using small spoon. Serve before a meal with toasted bread fingers or dark Dutch rye bread (pumpernickel) cut in long fingers.

Coleslaw

1 cup finely shredded cabbage
½ cup finely chopped celery
½ cup grated carrots
4 shallots, finely chopped
1 green apple, grated, or
½ cup finely chopped pineapple
1–2 tablespoons soya mayonnaise

Mix ingredients thoroughly.

Red cabbage salad

1 cup shredded red cabbage
½ cup finely chopped celery
4 shallots, finely chopped
1 green apple, grated
1–2 tablespoons soya mayonnaise

Mix ingredients together.

Spinach salad

$1\frac{1}{2}$ cups finely shredded Chinese cabbage
1 green apple, grated
1 cup finely shredded spinach
1–2 tablespoons of cold pressed oil
squeeze of lemon juice

Mix ingredients together.

Cauliflower salad

¼ medium cauliflower
2 cups diced Granny Smith apples
¼ cup finely chopped parsley
2 tablespoons yoghurt or sour cream
¼ cup chopped walnuts

Remove hard stem off cauliflower. Wash and break into small pieces or slice thinly. Mix with the diced apple, walnuts, parsley and yoghurt or sour cream. Serve on torn lettuce leaves and decorate with radishes or tomato quarters.

Carrot salad

1 cup grated carrot
1 green apple, grated
¼ cup finely chopped celery
4 shallots, finely chopped
2–3 tablespoons ground sesame seeds
1–2 tablespoons cold pressed oil

Mix ingredients together.

Zucchini salad

1 cup chopped zucchini
1 tomato, chopped
4 shallots, chopped
squeeze of lemon juice
2 tablespoons cold pressed oil

Mix ingredients together thoroughly. Serve with goat's or cottage cheese and Greek black olives.

Radish salad

lettuce or endive, finely shredded
3 radish, finely chopped
4 shallots, finely chopped
squeeze of lemon juice
1–2 tablespoons cold pressed oil

Mix ingredients together thoroughly.

Green bean salad

1 cup sliced cucumber
½ cup sliced green beans
2 cloves garlic crushed
4 shallots, finely chopped
2–3 tablespoons yoghurt

Mix together with sufficient yoghurt to coat ingredients.

Butternut pumpkin salad

1 cup finely grated butternut
½ cup walnut pieces
4 shallots, finely chopped
¼ cup chopped parsley
1 cup mixed bean sprouts or watercress
1–2 tablespoons cold pressed oil
1–2 radishes, sliced

Butternut should be grated very finely. Mix with walnut pieces, shallots, parsley and oil. Put mixture on a salad platter. Use sprouts or watercress to garnish by forming a ring around the edge of platter. Decorate with slices or radish.

Waldorf salad

1 cup finely chopped celery
2 green apples, finely diced
1 cup chopped walnuts
¼ cup cottage cheese
2–3 tablespoons yoghurt

Mix ingredients together.

Asparagus salad

12 asparagus spears
½ cup shredded Chinese cabbage
½ cup finely chopped celery
4 shallots, finely chopped
1 tablespoon soya mayonnaise
1–2 tomatoes, sliced
½ cup olives

Arrange asparagus spears on platter like spokes of a wheel. Mix cabbage, celery and shallots with mayonnaise. Fill in between spokes. Decorate with tomato slices around edge of platter, retaining some tomato slices to place in middle together with olives.

Tomato salad

1 cup chopped tomato (unsprayed if possible)
½ cup chopped cucumber
4 shallots, chopped
2 tablespoons chopped fresh basil
¼ cup sour cream or yoghurt

Mix ingredients together with either sour cream or yoghurt.

Beetroot salad

1 cup grated raw beetroot
½ cup finely chopped celery
4 shallots, finely chopped
1 medium-sized Granny Smith apple, grated
sour cream, for serving

Mix ingredients together and serve with sour cream.

Rice salad

2 cups cooked unpolished rice
1 medium-sized carrot, grated
½ cup chopped celery
½ cup chopped capsicum
5 gherkins, finely chopped
2–3 cups cubed fresh pineapple
¼ cup chopped shallots or chives
2 tablespoons fresh basil, chopped or 1 tablespoon dried basil
2 teaspoon ground coriander seeds
lettuce leaves, for serving
1–2 tomatoes, for decorating
olives, for decorating
parsley sprigs, for decorating

Mix ingredients together. Serve on bed of torn lettuce pieces. Decorate according to taste with sliced tomatoes, olives and parsley.

Swede or parsnip salad

1 cup finely grated swede or parsnip
4–5 shallots, chopped
½ cup chopped celery
¼ cup continental parsley
1–2 tablespoons cold pressed oil
lettuce leaves, for serving

Mix ingredients together thoroughly Serve on platter with lettuce leaves.

Potato salad

2 cups cubed cooked potatoes
¼ cup shallots or chives
3 gherkins
1 teaspoon dried basil
sour cream, to coat

Mix ingredients together thoroughly.

Note: Boiled eggs may be added too.

Salmon toss

1 large (220 g/8 oz) tin salmon, drained and flaked
1 cucumber, sliced
1 cup chopped celery
¼ cup chopped spring onions
1 tablespoon soya mayonnaise
seasoning to taste
lettuce
tomatoes (unsprayed if possible), cut in wedges

Combine salmon, cucumber, celery and spring onions. Pour mayonnaise over and toss lightly. Season and chill. Serve on a lettuce lined platter and garnish with tomato wedges.

Fish salad

1 cup flaked fish
1 cup cooked rice
1 small Granny Smith apple
1–2 gherkins
½ teaspoon (or to taste) horseradish paste or grated horseradish
vegetable salt, if necessary
1 teaspoon paprika
2–3 tablespoons soya mayonnaise
lettuce leaves, for serving

Mix fish and rice. Finely chop apple and gherkins and stir through the fish together with horseradish, salt, paprika and mayonnaise. Serve on a bed of torn lettuce pieces.

Fish dishes

Spicy crumbed sea fish

2 teaspoons coriander
½ teaspoon ginger
½ cup wheat germ
4 fish fillets
1 egg lightly beaten with 1 tablespoon cold pressed oil
cold pressed oil, for shallow frying
shallots, for garnishing
vegetable salt to taste
soya flour

Combine spices and wheat germ. Flour fillets and dip in beaten egg. Coat in spicy crumb mixture and shallow fry till golden. Serve straight from pan. Garnish with shallots.

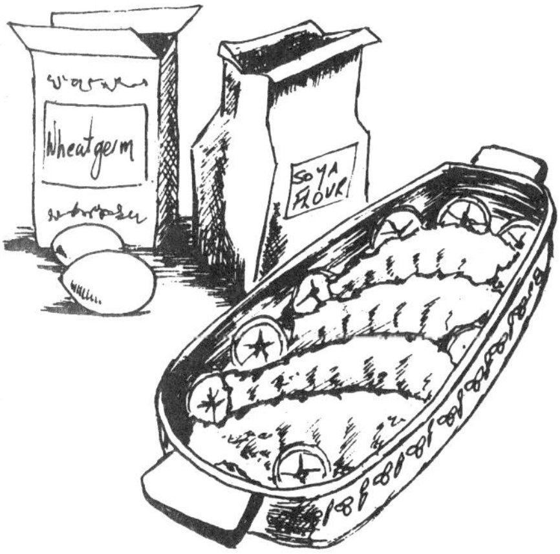

Fish rissoles

1 large tin salmon, drained and flaked
1 small onion, finely chopped
2 tablespoons finely chopped parsley
1 cup mashed potato
little salt
1 teaspoon water
approximately 1/4 cup wheat germ
cold pressed oil, for frying
1/2 teaspoon basil
1 egg
2 tablespoons soya or goat's milk

Mix fish with potato, onion, parsley, basil and a little salt. Beat egg with water. Add half to mixture; mix the other half with the milk. Shape rissoles. (A 1/4-cup flat measuring cup dipped in cold water, then filled with mixture makes nice shapes.) Dip rissoles in egg and milk mixture, then roll through wheat germ and fry both sides on hot oil showing slight vapour.

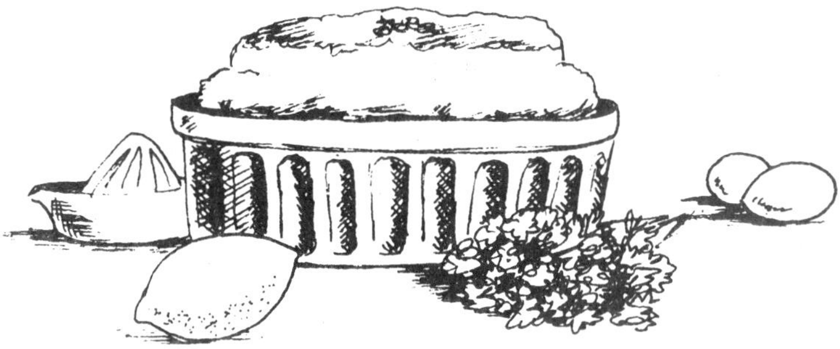

Marinated grilled fish

4 fish fillets

Marinade

2 cloves garlic, crushed
2 cm piece green ginger, finely grated
2 tablespoons Massel seasoning to taste
1 tablespoon lemon juice
1/2 cup fish or chicken stock

Combine all marinade ingredients and soak fillets in marinade for at least 1/2 hour. Place fillets on grill plate and baste with remainder of marinade while cooking.

Oven-baked fish cakes

1 egg
2 cups flaked fish (could be leftovers)
1cup cooked rice
1 onion, finely chopped
3 tablespoons cold pressed oil
squeeze of lemon juice
vegetable salt, if necessary
1 cup finely ground nuts or sunflower kernels

Beat egg and add all ingredients, except the nuts. Mix thoroughly. Shape into patties (best to use ½ a cup flat measuring cup rinsed in cold water). Roll through nuts and place on oiled baking sheet. Bake in 180°C oven until brown, about 20 minutes. Serve hot, garnished with sprigs of parsley.

Oven-baked bream

4 medium fillets of bream
generous pinch cayenne pepper
2 teaspoons basil
vegetable salt to taste
1 teaspoon thyme
lemon juice
¼ cup goat's milk
2 VitaBrits or approx. ¼ cup wheat germ or sesame seeds
1 tablespoon cold pressed oil

Grease small casserole dish; put in 2 fillets. Spread with half the cayenne pepper, then half the herbs. Repeat procedure with another layer of 2 fillets. Then sprinkle with lemon juice and milk. Put crushed VitaBrits, wheat germ or sesame seeds on top. Sprinkle the cold pressed oil over it and bake in 180°C oven for 30 minutes.

Salmon or tuna pie

1 large tin salmon or tuna, drained and flaked
1–2 tomatoes (unsprayed if possible), chopped
2 tablespoons finely chopped continental parsley
1 cup cooked rice
1 teaspoon dried basil
pinch vegetable salt, if necessary
1 tablespoon cold pressed oil
1 egg (optional)
pinch cayenne pepper
approximately ¼ cup wheat germ or sesame seeds

Mix all ingredients, except wheat germ and oil thoroughly. Put into greased casserole dish. Cover top with wheat germ or sesame seeds and sprinkle with cold pressed oil. Bake in 180°C oven for 30 minutes.

Salmon soufflé

2 tablespoons goat's or soya milk
2 tablespoons cold pressed oil
1 cup hot mashed potatoes
2 eggs
1 cup mashed salmon
1 tablespoon chopped parsley
vegetable salt, if necessary
1 teaspoon dried basil
pinch cayenne pepper
squeeze of lemon juice

Warm milk and oil and thoroughly mix potatoes into liquids while heating. Separate eggs and beat yolks into potato mixture. Stir in fish, parsley, salt, basil, cayenne pepper and lemon juice. Beat egg whites stiffly and fold lightly into mixture. Pour into well greased casserole and bake in 200°C oven until risen and golden brown. Sprinkle parsley on top.

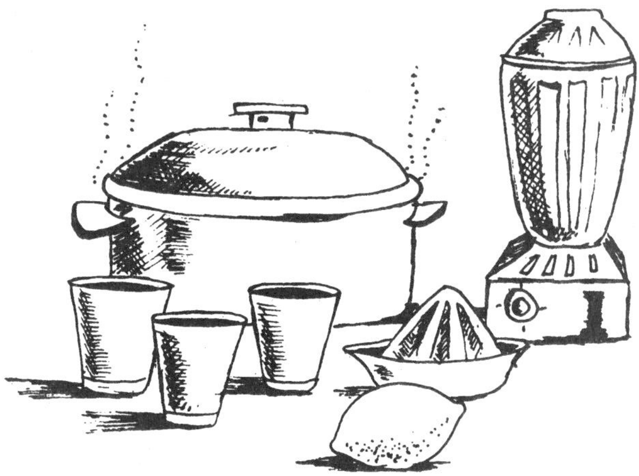

Protein dishes

How to make soya cream

Soak 1 cup of soya beans for 24 hours in cold water. Bring soya beans to the boil in saucepan while covered with water. Boil 30 minutes. Place boiling hot beans and about 2 cups of bean water or boiling water in electric blender. Add 3 tablespoons of vegetable oil and a little lemon juice. If necessary put cloth over blender to prevent hot liquid from spurting out. Turn control off and on to take up the heat. Blend for a few minutes until mixture is very fine and thick. Pour into paper cups and freeze until needed.

Note on cooking beans

Beans should be soaked 24 hours prior to cooking them. Soya beans take about 7 hours to cook, or can be cooked overnight in a crockpot on hot for 10 hours. Other beans take between 2–3 hours to cook, or about 4 hours in a crockpot.

Savoury roast

1 cup soya cream or mashed cooked soya beans
½ cup corn (optional)
1 medium-sized onion, chopped
½ cup chopped parsley
½ teaspoon salt (optional)
¼ teaspoon mixed herbs or bouquet garni
1 teaspoon paprika
½ cup chopped celery
1¼ cups cooked rice
Massel seasoning to taste
1 egg
approximately ¼ cup sesame seeds

Mix all ingredients, except last two, spoon into greased casserole dish and sprinkle with sesame seeds and paprika. Bake for 45 minutes until golden brown.

Soya cream rice loaf

2 eggs (1 hard boiled, 1 beaten)
1 large onion
½ cup celery
1 cup soya cream
1 teaspoon cold pressed oil
1 cup wheat germ
1 small tomato
1 cup rice
Massel seasoning to taste
vegetable salt to taste

Finely dice all ingredients and put into a greased casserole dish. Bake for 20–30 minutes in oven at 180°C.

Vegetarian loaf

2 cups cooked red beans
4 tablespoons cold pressed oil
1 green pepper, finely chopped
½ cup goat's or soya milk
1 cup finely chopped walnuts
½ teaspoon celery seeds
2 cups cooked rice
Massel seasoning to taste
2 eggs, lightly beaten or 2 rounded teaspoons Orgran egg replacer and 2 tablespoons water

Combine all ingredients and mix well. Turn onto a lightly oiled shallow baking pan and pat into a loaf. Bake in preheated 175°C oven for 30 minutes.

Vegetable pie

2 cups cooked haricot beans
1 onion, thinly sliced
1 turnip, grated
1carrot, grated
1 stick celery thinly sliced
1egg, beaten, or 1 rounded teaspoon Orgran egg replacer and 2 tablespoons water
Massel seasoning to taste
¼ cup cubed savoury roast or beef-flavoured TVP (soak in hot water for 15 minutes)
vegetable salt to taste
1 teaspoon dried basil

Mix beans with TVP or Savoury Roast, onion, turnip, celery and carrot with a small amount of vegetable stock or water. Add egg or egg replacer and seasoning and put into a greased casserole dish and cover with wheat germ or sesame seeds and dobs of butter. Bake at 180°C for 20–30 minutes.

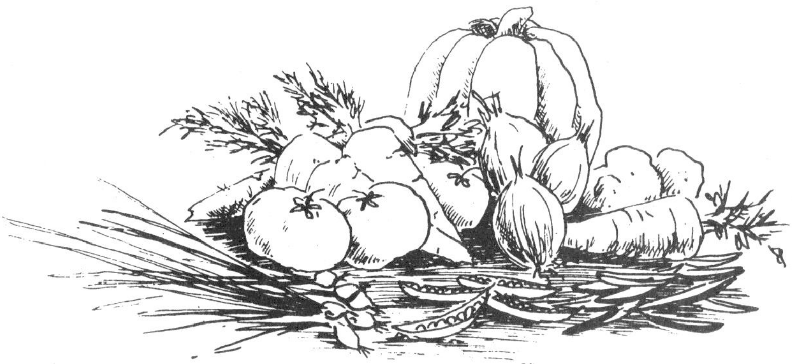

Saluggia bean stew

1 cup saluggia or brown beans
1 large onion
1 capsicum
1–2 eggs, beaten, or 1 rounded teaspoon Orgran egg replacer and 2 tablespoons water
pinch cayenne pepper
2 cloves
1 small bay leaf
vegetable salt to taste
cold pressed oil, for frying

Soak beans for 24 hours then cook until soft. Chop onion and capsicum, then sauté onion in oil until onion is transparent, about 5 minutes. Add bay leaf and cloves. Simmer for about 10 minutes, then add beans, egg, cayenne pepper and salt. Cook for another 5 minutes.

Kidney bean or brown bean croquettes

1 cup kidney beans or brown beans
3 medium-sized cooked potatoes, mashed
1 onion, chopped finely
pinch cayenne pepper
1 teaspoon Massel seasoning
1 egg
1–1½ cups wheat germ
cold pressed oil, for frying
parsley sprigs, for serving

Cook beans until soft and drain in colander. Vitamise or mash with a fork until fine. Mix beans with mashed potatoes. Sauté onion in oil until browned, then add to mixture together with cayenne pepper, Massel seasoning and salt. Mix thoroughly. Form either round or sausage-like rolls.

Beat egg with a little water. Roll croquettes first through wheat germ, then through beaten egg and through the wheat germ again. Fry in deep oil until brown and crisp. Drain on grease-proof paper. Serve with parsley.

Barlotti or kidney bean loaf

2 cups kidney or barlotti beans
1 bay leaf
3 cloves
1 tablespoon cold pressed oil
1 onion, finely chopped
¾ cup carrots, grated
¾ cup parsnips, grated
1 egg, beaten
1 level teaspoon Massel seasoning
vegetable salt (optional)

Cook beans with bay leaf and cloves until soft. Drain, add oil and other ingredients, combine well and cook in casserole dish in oven at 180 °C.

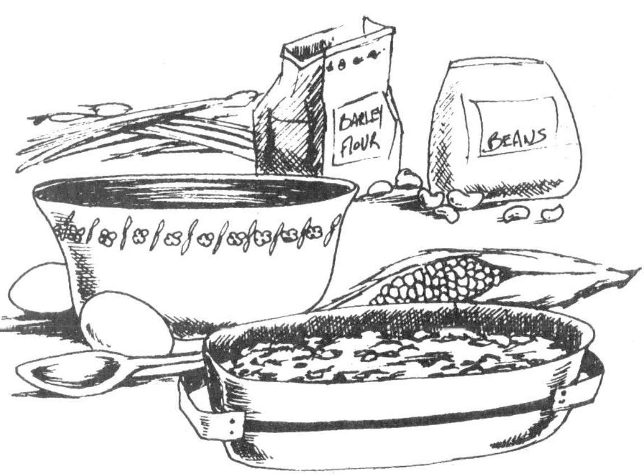

Chick pea casserole

1 cup chick peas
1 cup spinach, chopped
1 onion
1 tablespoon cold pressed oil
1 clove garlic, finely crushed
¼ cup chopped red capsicum
1 tomato, chopped
½ teaspoon ground ginger
2 cloves
1 egg, beaten
2 tablespoons rice flour
Massel seasoning to taste

Soak chick peas in water for 24 hours, then cook until soft. Chop onion. Heat oil in frying pan. Sauté onion, garlic and capsicum for a few minutes. Then add spinach and tomato and simmer for a few minutes with ginger and cloves. Add all other ingredients and mix together. Put in oiled casserole dish. Bake in 180°C oven for 20–30 minutes.

Lima and green bean dish

2 eggs or 2 rounded teaspoons Orgran egg replacer and 4 tablespoons water
½ cup chopped shallots
1 cup cooked lima beans
1 cup slightly cooked green beans
½ cup corn (optional)
2 tablespoons chopped nuts
¼ cup beef-flavoured TVP (soak in hot water for 15 min)
2 tablespoons maize or barley flour
vegetable salt to taste
¼ cup wheat germ
little cold pressed oil

Beat eggs or prepare egg replacer, then add shallots and cooked beans. Add all other ingredients and put in oiled casserole dish. Top with wheat germ and sprinkle a little cold pressed oil on top. Cook in 175–200°C oven for 20 minutes.

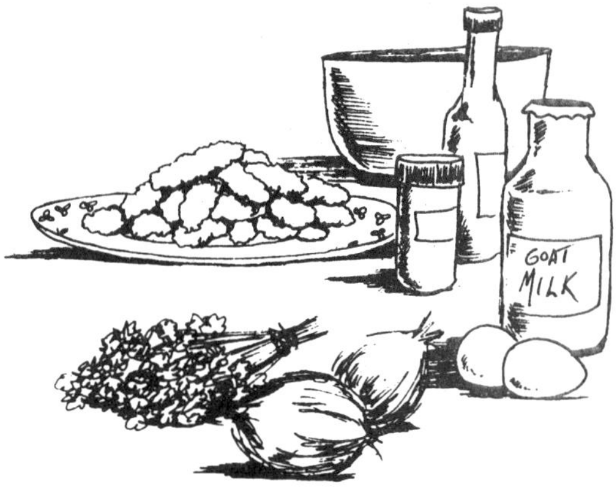

Cannelini bean croquettes

1 cup cannelini beans
1–2 onions
3 medium-sized cooked potatoes
½ cup chopped parsley
1 teaspoon Massel seasoning
½ teaspoon turmeric
½ teaspoon paprika
cayenne pepper, as required
1 egg
1 teaspoon goat's milk
1–1½ cups wheat germ
cold pressed oil, for frying
parsley sprigs, for serving

Cook the beans until soft. Chop onions and sauté until slightly browned. Mash beans and potatoes and mix with onions, parsley, Massel seasoning, turmeric, paprika, cayenne pepper and salt. Knead and make into balls. Slightly flatten balls. Beat egg together with the milk. Put the croquettes through this first and then through the wheat germ. Fry in hot oil until brown on each side. Serve with parsley.

Mung beans

1 cup mung beans
¾ litre (1¼ pints) water
Massel seasoning to taste
3 teaspoons cold pressed oil
1 onion, finely sliced
1 cup cubed Savoury Roast
or ¼ cup beef-flavoured TVP
(soak in hot water for 15 min)
1 teaspoon turmeric
1 teaspoon ground coriander

Soak mung beans overnight. Add Massel seasoning to soaking water, then cook until beans are just tender. Do not over-cook. Heat oil and gently sauté onions and Savoury Roast, if using, until onions transparent. Add to mung beans, retaining cooking liquid. If using TVP, add to mixture along with turmeric and coriander. Simmer without over-cooking beans. Add vegetable salt if necessary. Serve with rice.

Nut galantine

1 carrot
1 medium-sized onion
1 cup chopped mixed nuts
1 cup brown rice
2 tablespoons chopped parsley
1 tablespoon cold pressed oil
1 large egg, beaten, or 1 rounded teaspoon
Orgran egg replacer and 2 tablespoons water

Grate carrot and chop onion, then mix together with nuts, rice and parsley. Add oil and bind with beaten egg or egg replacer. Press mixture into a well greased savoury roll jar and steam for about 2½ hours.

Lentil roast

1 cup brown lentils
1 egg
1 onion, grated or finely chopped
2 tablespoons chopped parsley
1 medium-sized carrot, grated
pinch thyme
1 cup goat's milk
¼ cup tahini
1 teaspoon vegetable salt (opt)
½ cup rolled oats or rice
approx. ¼ cup sesame seeds

Cook lentils until soft, about 20 minutes. Break egg into bowl and mix with onion, parsley carrot, thyme, milk, tahini and salt. Mix well, then add lentils and rolled oats. Pour mixture into greased casserole dish, sprinkle whole sesame seeds on top and bake in 175°C oven for 30–45 minutes.

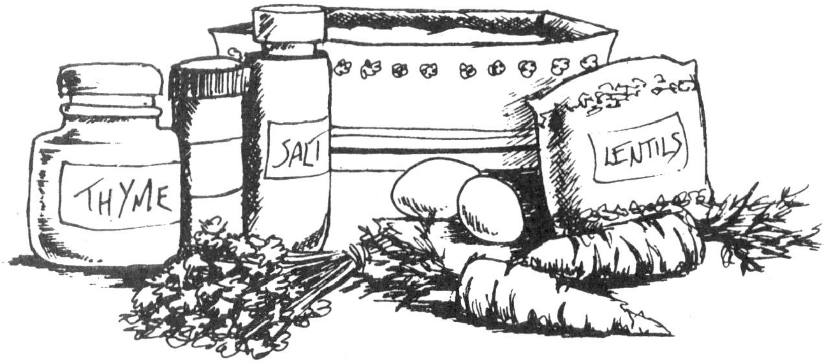

Lentil or split pea patties

1 cup lentils or split peas
½ cup TVP mince (optional)
1 egg
¼ teaspoon thyme
½ teaspoon turmeric
½ teaspoon vegetable salt
1 small onion, finely chopped
rolled oats or rolled barley
cold pressed oil, for frying

Just cover lentils with water and cook until soft, about 15 minutes. Just cover TVP in boiling water for 10 minutes. Beat egg in bowl and add thyme, turmeric and salt, then onion, lentils and TVP. Stir thoroughly and add sufficient rolled oats to make a fairly solid consistency. Heat oil in frying pan (just enough oil to cover frying pan bottom). Take a tablespoonful of mixture and form patties while putting them in the pan. Flatten them slightly with a fork when in the pan. Fry until golden brown on both sides.

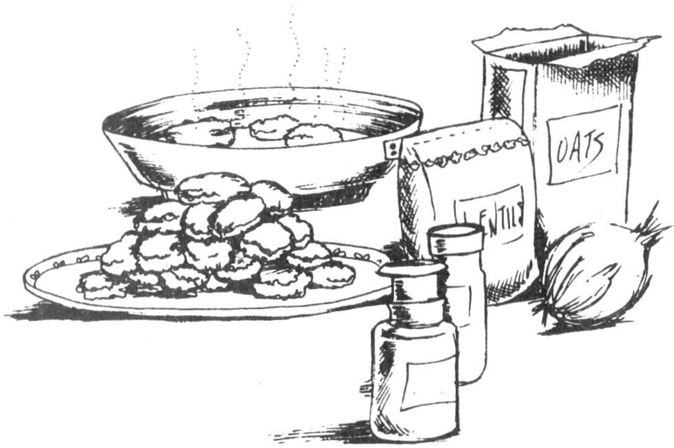

Split pea roast

2 cups split peas
3 cups water
½ cup crumbled tofu
1/2 cup leftover vegetable loaf or other loaf
1 medium-sized carrot, grated
1 large onion, grated
1 cup chopped leeks
1 teaspoon dried basil
pinch cayenne
1 egg, beaten
1 teaspoon Massel seasoning

Soak split peas overnight in water, then cook until soft. Mix together thoroughly with other ingredients. Bake in 175 °C oven until set. Serve hot with mint sauce and vegetables, cold on salad, or as a sandwich filling.

Sunflower seed loaf

1 ½ cups ground sunflower seeds
1 cup cooked lentils
½ cup chopped walnuts
½ cup grated raw beetroot
¾ cup finely ground sesame seed meal
3 tablespoons minced chives or shallots
2 eggs, beaten slightly or 2 rounded teaspoons Orgran egg replacer and
4 tablespoons water
2 tablespoons lemon juice
½ cup diced celery
½ cup cooked buckwheat or brown rice
Massel seasoning to taste
1 tablespoon cold pressed oil

Blend together all ingredients, and press into an oiled baking dish. Bake at 170 °C until done – about 60 minutes. Serve hot from the oven with a raw salad.

Savoury nut casserole

3 small eggs
1 tablespoon goat's milk or soya milk
2 heaped tablespoons finely chopped walnuts
2 medium-sized onions, finely chopped
1 tablespoon finely chopped parsley or celery leaves
1 cup cooked rice
1 cup cubed marinated tofu
1–2 teaspoons dried sweet basil
pinch mixed herbs
vegetable salt to taste
approximately $\frac{1}{4}$ cup sesame seeds

Beat eggs with goat's or soya milk. Mix all ingredients except sesame seeds together and place in a greased casserole dish. Top with sesame seeds. Bake in moderate oven (180°C) for 30–45 minutes.

Vegetables

Vegetables should not be peeled, but scrubbed only. By grating, dicing or slicing vegetables, such as carrots, beetroot, pumpkin, they cook much quicker and not so many valuable elements are lost.

The best ways to cook vegetables are baking in the oven, or the waterless way. The best utensils to use for cooking are stainless steel, enamel, Corning Ware, Pyrex and other ovenware. Never use aluminium cooking utensils. The aluminium is a poison which is absorbed by the food. It has a bad effect on the stomach and bowels, and deposits in the brain are linked to Alzheimer's disease.

Cooking vegetables at boiling temperature destroys both vitamins and enzymes, which are essential for proper digestion of your food. Cooking below boiling temperature as in waterless cooking and crock pots, retains the vitamins and other valuable nutrients. Waterless cooking is by far the best method. To be able to do this a stainless steel saucepan specially equipped for this way of cooking is required. Some even have a thermometer fitted into the lid with a red mark warning when the temperature is too high.

For waterless cooking, just cover the bottom of a saucepan with water and add a little oil. Place the clean vegetables in the saucepan on medium to high heat. When the lid starts to ride on the vapour, reduce the heat as low as possible (a flame distributor can be placed in between). Turn the lid so that it continues to ride on the vapour. If lid lifts up, temperature is still a little too high. Leave vegetables on this low temperature for the required cooking time. If you have a gas stove, a little more water may need to be added.

Do not add salt or soda to any fresh vegetables when cooking them. With the 'waterless cooking' method all natural salts, minerals and vitamins, as well as the flavour of the food, are retained.

To finish off and to enhance the flavour, add a little soft butter or a little yoghurt. Herbs or some harmless spices can also be added.

Approximate cooking times

beans, string, wax, fresh lima	15–20 minutes
beetroot, sliced; onions, whole	20–25 minutes
beetroot, grated; carrots, grated	10–15 minutes
broccoli; cauliflower; celery; kale	8–10 minutes
carrots, whole; small turnips; pumpkin with skin	20–25 minutes
corn; brussels sprouts	10–12 minutes
eggplant; leeks; capsicum; squash	8–10 minutes
greens; cabbage; tomatoes	3–5 minutes
onions, sliced; fresh peas	5–8 minutes
parsnips, sliced	10–15 minutes
potatoes, sweet	20–35 minutes
potatoes, small or halves	30–35 minutes

Carrots

Scrub carrots, cut into slices or fingers 5 cm (2") long. Waterless cook with a teaspoon of cold pressed safflower or sunflower oil until cooked. Top with finely chopped parsley.

Parsnips

Cook in the same way as carrots.

Green beans

Take threads off beans, break in two or three pieces. Wash beans and waterless cook. Top with a little nutmeg.

Peas

Shell peas and waterless cook. Top with chopped parsley or mint.

Snow peas or sugar snap peas

Do not shell. Thread peas and waterless cook. No need for any topping. Can be served with a little soft butter when on low allergy diet.

Baby carrots and sugar snap peas

Wash and scrub carrots and waterless cook with a little soft butter Add the threaded sugar peas when carrots are half cooked. Top with finely chopped parsley when serving.

Pumpkin

Cut pumpkin in cubes, skin included, and waterless cook. Top with chopped parsley or watercress. If cooked in oven, cut in large pieces or even bake the whole pumpkin. Oil baking dish with cold pressed oil.

Endive

Prepare as spinach. Add some grated Granny Smith apple.

Beetroot

Wash and scrub beets. Cut into thin slices or coarsely grate. Waterless cook. Fry one finely chopped onion in cold pressed safflower oil until transparent. Add to cooked beetroot. Also add a little lemon juice.

Swedes

Wash and scrub the skin. Waterless cook. After swedes are soft simmer in sauce (see cauliflower sauce recipe below). Dust with a little nutmeg when serving.

Sweetcorn

Simmer in 2 cm water for about 15 minutes. Serve with yoghurt or light sour cream.

Spinach

Wash and chop spinach and waterless cook. Mix with a little yoghurt or light sour cream.

Cauliflower

Divide cauliflower into even pieces. Take off hard stalks. Put in water and vegetable salt for about 15 minutes. Then place in saucepan with stalks down and waterless cook.

Make a sauce using ½ cup goat's milk, 1 tablespoon rice flour and 1 teaspoon cummin seed or chopped parsley. Add flour to cold milk and bring to the boil while stirring with French whisk. Reduce heat and add cummin or parsley, continuing to stir until thickened.

Pour over cauliflower when serving. Dust with nutmeg, but only if no cummin seed is used.

Broccoli

Divide broccoli in pieces. Take off hard stalks. Waterless cook and serve with a little soft butter.

White or savoy cabbage

Clean and shred cabbage. Waterless cook with a little cold pressed oil and caraway seeds (to avoid flatulence). Add a cored, diced Granny Smith apple to reduce the cabbage smell.

Brussels sprouts

Cook as white cabbage, but leave out the diced apple.

Witlof

Method 1 – Cook witlof whole in a little fresh goat's milk (or rice milk) until soft. Take out witlof and add a little soft butter to milk. Add rice or barley flour to thicken. Now add witlof to the sauce and stir around.

Method 2 – Cut witlof in 2 cm pieces. Cook with a little water and soft butter until soft. Add a little soy sauce and Parmesan cheese. Thicken with rice or barley flour.

Red cabbage with Granny Smith apples

Wash and core one large Granny Smith apple. Cut into small pieces and waterless cook. Wash and shred the cabbage. Add to cooked apples with 1 bay leaf and 2 cloves.

When both apples and cabbage are soft, mix thoroughly. Thicken fluid with arrowroot. Add a little lemon juice.

Leeks or onions

Remove any dry, dirty leaves. Cut leeks into 2 cm (¾") pieces, including green parts. Wash very thoroughly in a lot of water. Strain, then place in saucepan and waterless cook. Onions should be cooked in the same way, using either very small onions or onion quarters with larger onions. Add a little lemon juice when cooked.

Make a sauce from ½ cup goat's milk and 1 tablespoon rice flour using the method described for cauliflower sauce. Add to leeks and simmer for a few minutes.

Jerusalem artichokes

Wash and scrub artichokes, taking out any bad parts. Cut into 4 cm (1½") pieces. Waterless cook. Simmer in sauce the same as that prepared for leeks.

Globe artichokes

These contain the biochemical inulin, which is important in restoring the bowel wall.

With stainless steel knife slice off stem. Remove the coarse outer leaves. Cut off top ⅓ of the globe and any thorny tips. Rinse thoroughly with lukewarm water, rub with lemon. Place in stainless steel saucepan, globe down in 2 cm of water. Cook for 20–30 minutes until tender. Add a little butter.

Vegetable mould

1 cup diced mixed vegetables such as carrot, pumpkin, beetroot, parsley, beans or peas, zucchini, choko, squash, shallots or onions
½ cup of water
½ cup of vegetable juice
1 rounded teaspoon agar agar

Waterless cook vegetables until just tender. Heat water until at boiling point, add juice, then bring to boil again. Stir in agar for one minute. Pour a little into mould rinsed with cold water. Add vegetables and pour in remaining agar mixture. Mix vegetables and agar mixture with spoon, leave to cool, then put in fridge and turn out of mould onto a plate.

Beetroot mould

3 cups cubed cooked beetroot
2 cups water, including juice of beetroot
3 rounded teaspoons agar agar
juice of 1 lemon

Heat water and juice to boiling point, add agar and lemon juice, stir and take off heat. Rinse mould with cold water, put some agar mixture in mould, add the beetroot then fill up with agar mixture. Cool and turn out of mould onto plate.

Note: If preferred, use individual moulds for each person rather than one large mould.

Ratatouille

2 large onions
2 capsicums (1 red, 1 green)
1 eggplant
4 zucchini
3 ripe tomatoes (unsprayed if possible), peeled
1 tablespoon chopped fresh basil
1 tablespoon chopped fresh oregano
pinch cayenne pepper
2 tablespoons chopped fresh parsley
1–2 tablespoons cold pressed oil

Cut vegetables in slices or bite-size pieces. Heat oil and saute onion until transparent, add capsicum, eggplant, zucchini and tomatoes. Simmer for 30 minutes or desired time. Add herbs.

Stir-fried vegetable dish

2 tablespoons cold pressed oil
1 cup sliced onions
1 cup sliced beans
1 cup sliced carrots
1 cup sliced celery
1 clove garlic, crushed/chopped
a little Massel seasoning
1 cup water
2 teaspoons arrowroot blended in a little water

Heat oil in heavy frying pan. Put in all vegetables, adding celery last. Stir for a few minutes, then add Massel seasoning and water. Cover and simmer for 5 minutes, then add arrowroot while stirring. Serve at once.

Staple dishes

By staple dishes we mean such foods as potatoes, rice, buckwheat and pasta, even whole millet can be used as such.

Potatoes can be cooked in a saucepan or baked in their jackets. Before cooking, scrub with a brush and take out any bad spots. Green potatoes must not be used. When cooked in a saucepan, pour off any water left after potatoes are soft and put back on element for a few minutes until potatoes are dry and floury If potatoes are baked, they take about an hour in a moderate oven.

A variety of recipes for preparing potatoes are provided in this section. Alternatively rice can be eaten, either as is or using the recipes provided.

Potato casserole

1 onion, chopped
2 tablespoons cold pressed oil
1 teaspoon turmeric
½ teaspoon sweet basil
½ teaspoon chervil
¼ teaspoon coriander
½ cup finely chopped celery or chives and parsley mixed
½ teaspoon vegetable salt
2 tablespoons rice flour
2 cups water
Massel seasoning
3 cups diced cooked potatoes

Sauté onion in oil until beginning to brown. Add turmeric, sweet basil, chervil, coriander, celery or chives and parsley, salt, and stir well. Add rice flour and water mixed with Massel seasoning. Stir until thickened. Add potatoes, then place mixture in casserole dish. Bake in oven at 180°C for 20–30 minutes.

Potato hotpot with lettuce

4 medium potatoes
1 onion
1 tablespoon cold pressed oil
¼ cup goat's milk
a little vegetable salt
1 cup cooked haricot beans
2 cups shredded lettuce leaves

Cook potatoes in about ½ cup water. Chop onion and fry in oil. Add to potatoes and mash together, adding milk, salt and beans. Lastly add shredded lettuce leaves.

Hutspot

4 medium potatoes
1 cup diced carrots
1 large onion
1 tablespoon cold pressed oil
¼ cup goat's milk
Massel seasoning to taste
vegetable salt, if required

Cook potatoes and carrots together in about ½ cup water Chop onion and fry in oil. Add to potatoes and mash together with the milk, Massel seasoning and salt. Serve as it is or put in a casserole dish, make lines with a fork and brown for about 10 minutes in the oven.

Spiced potatoes

2 tablespoons cold pressed oil
1 tomato, finely chopped
4 tablespoons green pepper, diced
¼ teaspoon cayenne pepper
¼ teaspoon ground turmeric
¼ teaspoon ground allspice
¼ teaspoon ground ginger
¼ teaspoon vegetable salt
½ teaspoon ground coriander
5 large cooked potatoes, diced

Heat oil in a large heavy frying pan over a moderate heat. Add tomato, green pepper, cayenne pepper, turmeric, allspice, ginger, salt and coriander. Cook, stirring constantly, for 2 minutes. Add potatoes and cook, stirring until potatoes are coated with spices and heated through.

Potato pancakes

4 large potatoes, grated
2 eggs or 1 rounded teaspoon Orgran egg replacer and 2 tablespoons water
½ cup cornmeal or buckwheat flour
vegetable salt to taste
pinch cayenne pepper
2 tablespoons parsley finely chopped
cold pressed oil, for frying
1 teaspoon dried basil

Put raw grated potatoes into a basin, then mix two unbeaten eggs or egg replacer, cornmeal or flour, salt, pepper, parsley and basil into the potatoes. When thoroughly mixed, drop tablespoons full of mixture into a pan with very hot oil and fry until a light brown on both sides.

Rice and curry dish

2 cups brown rice or barley (soaked in water overnight)
3 cups water
1 teaspoon cold pressed oil
1 tablespoon dried basil
vegetable salt to taste
1 large onion, chopped
1½ cups chopped celery
½ cup chopped choko
½ cup green bean pieces
1 tomato, chopped
2 cups savoury roast or ½ cup beef-flavoured TVP (soak in hot water for 15 min)
2 teaspoons mild curry
3 tablespoons yoghurt

Bring rice to boil in water with oil. Simmer for about 1 hour. Add basil and a little vegetable salt.

Curry mixture

Fry onion in a little cold pressed oil and add vegetables and Savoury Roast or TVP, then curry. Lastly add yoghurt.

Barley and spinach pasta

250 g (9 oz) barley and spinach pasta
2 cups water
1 tablespoon cold pressed oil
1 onion, chopped
2 cloves garlic crushed
2 tomatoes (unsprayed if possible), chopped
Massel seasoning to taste
3 tablespoons yoghurt or light sour cream

Bring water to boil first, then add pasta and cook for about 5 minutes. Drain. Heat oil and sauté onions and garlic until soft, then add tomatoes and Massel seasoning. Before serving stir yoghurt or sour cream through pasta.

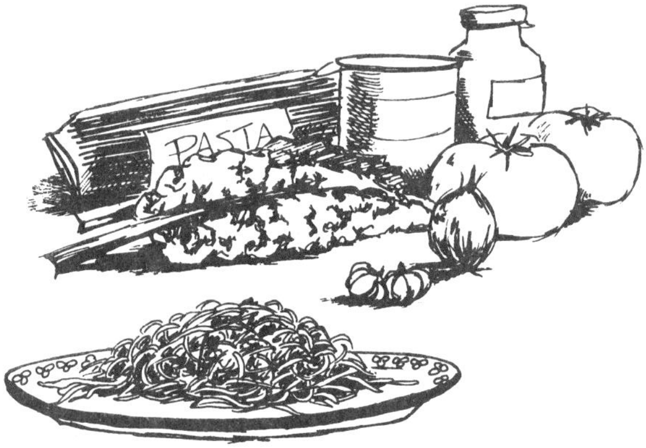

Savoury millet

1 1/4 cups hulled millet
3 cups water
1 tablespoon grapeseed oil
1 large onion
1 cup chopped celery
1 cup peas
1 tomato, cubed
Massel seasoning to taste
cold pressed oil, for frying

Cook millet in water with the oil until soft. Chop onion and sauté with celery until onion transparent. Add to millet together with peas, tomato and Massel seasoning. Can be pressed into cakes and fried on both sides in a little oil.

Buckwheat Roast

1 cup buckwheat
1 large onion, chopped
1 tablespoon cold pressed oil
½ cup diced capsicum (optional)
1 cup diced celery
1 egg, beaten, or 1 rounded tablespoon Orgran egg replacer and 2 tablespoons water
Massel seasoning to taste

Boil buckwheat until cooked – about 10 minutes. Sauté onion in oil until slightly brown, then add capsicum and celery. Mix with cooked buckwheat. Stir in beaten egg or egg replacer and Massel seasoning if required. Put in oiled casserole dish and bake in oven at 180°C for about 15 minutes.

Note: Onion, celery and capsicum can be cooked together with buckwheat rather than frying. This is a better way for people with liver or gallbladder trouble.

Bami goreng (vegetarian Indonesian dish)

250 g (9 oz) spinach vermicelli
5 shallots bulbs or spring onions
3 garlic cloves, crushed
1 tablespoon cold pressed oil
1 cup diced celery
1 cup shredded cabbage
1 cup green beans, sliced
2 cups chopped leeks or spring onion tips
1 cup savoury roast or similar commercial product
1 teaspoon ginger powder
Massel seasoning to taste
juice of 1 lemon
vegetable salt to taste
2 eggs (optional)
1 tablespoon water (optional)
60–80 g (3 oz) olives

Boil vermicelli in a lot of water until cooked. Separate and drain in colander. Chop shallots or spring onions and saute with garlic in oil until slightly browned. Add celery, cabbage, beans, leeks and spring onion tips and saute another 10 minutes. Add Soyabean Roast and ginger powder. Leave for a few more minutes on low heat. Stir this mixture through the cooked vermicelli together with Massel seasoning and lemon juice. Simmer for about 10 minutes. Add salt.

Make omelette by beating eggs, then adding water and beating until frothy. Fry omelette on both sides until slightly brown, then cut into strips. Put Bami Goreng into serving dish and decorate with strips of omelette and olives.

Fried rice

1–2 tablespoons cold pressed oil
medium to large sized onion, chopped
3–4 cups cold cooked brown rice or barley (soaked in water overnight before cooking)
$\frac{1}{2}$–$\frac{2}{3}$ cup diced carrot, half cooked
$\frac{1}{4}$–$\frac{1}{2}$ cup diced red capsicum or chopped celery
1 cup peas
1 tablespoon Massel seasoning
a little vegetable salt
1 cup chopped shallots

Heat oil, sauté onion for a few minutes, then add rice. Break up lumps and stir to distribute oil evenly. Sauté a little longer to crisp the rice. Add vegetables and salt. When uniformly heated add Massel seasoning. Add shallots.

Optional ingredients

$\frac{1}{2}$ cup of any of the following: chopped water chestnuts, bamboo shoots, pineapple pieces, soya beans or chick peas, chopped up softly scrambled egg.

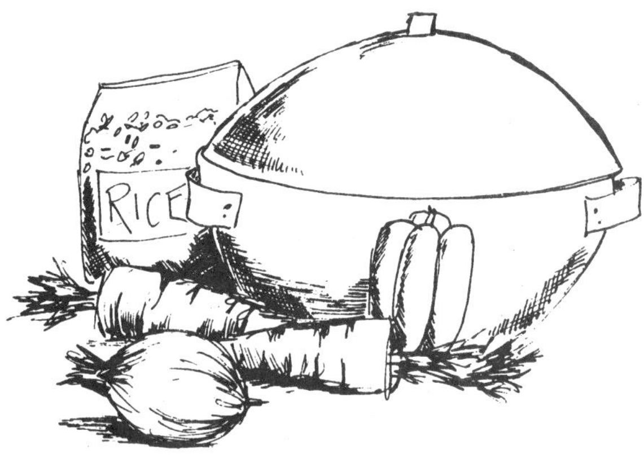

Grains and desserts

None of these recipes contain wheat, as this a food to which people are most allergic. For those who do not know, buckwheat is not wheat. If you are allergic to any of the grains, they can usually be substituted with one to which you are not allergic. There is a non-allergenic baking powder available at health food shops. The desserts contain some artificial sweetening. Be sure to buy the most natural type.

Important note

Orgran egg replacer can be used in place of eggs: 1 heaped teaspoon of egg Orgran mixed with 2 tablespoons of water is equivalent to one egg.

'Artificial sweetener' in the following recipes refers to Stevia. Stevia is made from a safe herb and is 30 times sweeter than sugar. Use carefully – it is best to make a liquid and add Stevia drop-by-drop while tasting.

Waffles (not gluten free)

Cashew-oat

2 1/4 cups water
1/2 cup wholemeal flour
1 cup rolled oats
1/2 cup raw cashews
1 tablespoon cold pressed oil
pinch vegetable salt (optional)

Multi-grain

2 1/4 cups water
1/2 cup rye flour
1/2 cup wholemeal flour
1/2 cup soya flour
1/2 cup rolled oats
1 tablespoon cold pressed oil
pinch vegetable salt (optional)

Gluten-free Waffles

2 1/4 cups water
1/2 cup millet meal
1/4 cup soya flour
1 1/2 cups buckwheat flour
1 tablespoon cold pressed oil
pinch vegetable salt (optional)

Combine all ingredients in electric blender until light and foamy. Let stand while waffle iron is heating. When red light turns off, put about 1/2 cup of mixture in waffle iron. (If not enough or too much, adjust with next waffle.) Do not open iron until waffle is cooked, about 8–10 minutes, when little or no steam escapes. If waffle is too thick and not crunchy add a little more water to mixture. Keep warm in low oven if necessary. Serve with tahini.

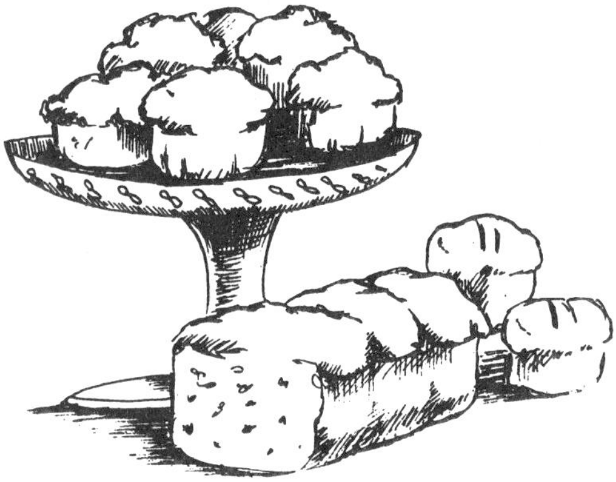

Yeast-free pancakes (gluten free)

2 eggs, beaten
1 cup buckwheat flour
½ litre (2 cups) goat's milk
2 tablespoons cold pressed oil (more if required)
little vegetable salt if necessary

Mix eggs into the flour and salt, gradually adding milk and 1 tablespoon oil. Heat 1 tablespoon oil in frying pan and make thin pancakes. Slightly brown on each side. Serve with tahini or fill with Savoury Filling and roll up.

Savoury filling

1 tablespoon cold pressed oil
1 medium onion, finely chopped
2 tablespoons rice flour
pinch vegetable salt
½ teaspoon sweet basil
1 cup well-cooked brown lentils
1 tablespoon chopped parsley

Heat oil in pan and cook onion. Stir in flour, salt, basil and lentils. Let mixture bubble. Gradually add milk, stirring all the time. Take from heat, then add parsley.

Pikelets (low gluten)

½ cup fine millet flour
½ cup fine barley flour
½ cup soya flour
1 tablespoon fine cornmeal
1 tablespoon ground linseed
1 tablespoon sunflower kernels or ground nuts
½ teaspoon cinnamon
300 ml (½ pint) water
2 teaspoons Orgran egg replacer and 4 tablespoons water
pinch vegetable salt
herbs to taste, if required
cold pressed oil, for frying

Mix ingredients and beat with electric beater if possible or use a whisk. Oil frying pan and heat until a light vapour appears. Drop in tablespoons full of mixture. Cover pan with lid. Fry both sides of pikelets until slightly browned, keeping lid on all the time at a medium temperature.

Serve when ready or put in containers lined with grease-proof paper. Put paper between layers to avoid pikelets sticking together.

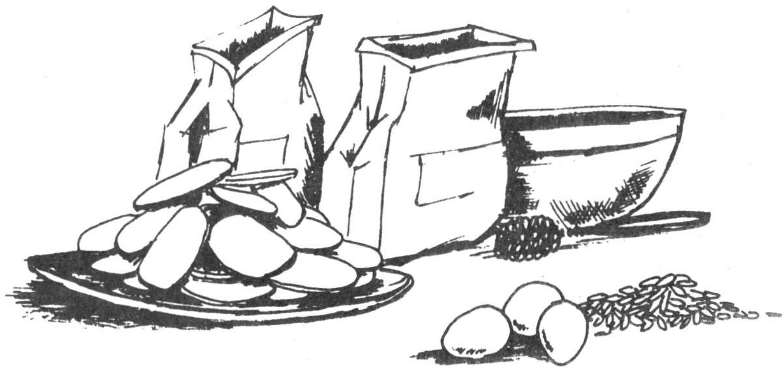

Cornmeal pancakes

1½ cups unrefined yellow cornmeal
½ teaspoon vegetable salt
2 cups goat s or soya milk
2 tablespoons cold pressed oil
1 egg yolk, slightly beaten
1 egg white, stiffly beaten

Stir together dry ingredients. Add milk, 1 tablespoon of oil, egg yolk, and fold in egg white. Drop spoonfuls of mixture into hot oiled pan, and cook until golden brown on both sides.

Corn bread cakes

1 cup unrefined yellow cornmeal
1½ cups boiling water
½ teaspoon vegetable salt
2 tablespoons cold pressed oil

Add cornmeal all at once to salted boiling water. Stir until it clings together in a ball, pulling away from the sides of the saucepan. Remove from the heat. Add oil and beat briskly. Place spoonfuls of mixture onto a lightly oiled tray and flatten with a fork. Bake at 200°C until nicely browned, about 30 minutes.

Tofu cream

300 g (10½ oz) tofu, drained
1 teaspoon vanilla essence
1–2 tablespoons honey or equivalent amount of sweetener
1 tablespoon water

Blend and whip all ingredients till creamy. Vanilla essence can be replaced with 1 teaspoon of almond essence or 1 tablespoon of coconut cream, depending on your allergies.

Stephen's carob cake

3 cups fine rice flour or fine cornmeal
3 teaspoons low allergy baking powder
2 eggs
125 g (4½ oz) soft butter
100 g (3½ oz) sugarless carob buds
2 tablespoons carob powder
½ teaspoon vanilla essence
½ cup milk and 1 cup water or 1½ cups water
artificial sweetening, equivalent to ¾ cup sugar

Line bottom of 20 cm (8") baking tin with grease-proof paper, then grease sides of tin and paper. Sift flour and mix in the baking powder. Cream soft butter with sweetener until fluffy. Add 1 egg first, or half the egg replacer, then beat well with electric beater or Bamix. Melt carob buds in small bowl above boiling water.

Mix milk and water, add half of this together with the melted carob buds to mixture, then beat again. Add half the flour, the carob powder and vanilla essence while beating. Now add the other egg or remaining egg replacer then the remaining milk and beat together with the remaining flour. Beat thoroughly and pour into the greased baking tin. Bake in 150°C oven for 50 minutes. Cool on rack. When cold cover with Tofu Cream, and decorate with almonds, hazelnuts or other nuts and pepitas.

Pumpkin pie

Pastry

150 g (5¼ oz) butter
½ cup arrowroot
1½ cups rice flour
1 teaspoon lemon juice

Work butter into flour and arrowroot with two knives, add lemon juice and mix into ingredients. Line pie plate with pastry moulding with hand.

Filling

500 g (1 lb) pumpkin
½ teaspoon each nutmeg, cinnamon and ginger
¼ teaspoon all spice
2 eggs or egg-replacer
sugar substitute equivalent to ¼ cup sugar
1 cup soya milk
3 tablespoons soya milk powder

Cook pumpkin, then add spices, eggs, sweetener and milks. Mix in blender until creamy. Place in pie shell, and cook at 200°C for 10 minutes, then at 180°C for 35 minutes.

Carob pudding (cold)

2 cups goat's milk
4 tablespoons rice flour
1 tablespoon arrowroot
4 tablespoons carob powder
sugar substitute equivalent to 2 tablespoons sugar

Mix ingredients and bring to boil while stirring with French whisk. Boil a few minutes while thickening. Rinse mould with cold water, then pour mixture into mould. Serve with cold custard or coconut cream.

Milk porridge

4 cups goat's milk or soya milk or 2 cups goat's milk and 2 cups water
4 rounded tablespoons millet meal
1 rounded tablespoon cornmeal
1 rounded tablespoon rice flour
1 rounded tablespoon soya flour (optional)

Combine all ingredients in a saucepan. Bring to nearly boiling, stirring constantly. Turn to a low heat and continue stirring for another ½ minute. Leave simmering with lid on until well cooked (approx. 20 minutes). If the porridge is too thick add more milk or water.

Custard

2 cups goat's milk
½ tablespoon arrowroot
2 teaspoons pure vanilla
1½ tablespoons (level) rice
2 eggs
sugar substitute equivalent to 1 tablespoon sugar

Mix all ingredients together, stirring with French whisk until thickened. Serve hot or cold.

Note: Do not replace eggs with egg replacer in this recipe.

Easy bread (gluten free)

1 cup fine rice flour
1 cup fine buckwheat flour
1 cup fine millet flour
2 eggs/egg substitute
1½ cups soya milk

Sift flours. Beat eggs, and add to flours. Stir in soya milk, and mix thoroughly. Put in greased loaf tin (24 x 10 cm/10" x 4"). Bake in 180°C oven for approximately 1½ hours.

Sour dough bread (not gluten free)

Sour dough (leavening agent)

Mix 1 cup of rye or whole wheat or millet flour with sufficient water to make a stiff dough. Cover and put in a warm place (30°C). Leave for 8 days, when the dough has developed a pleasant aroma. It is now ready to be used in bread making.

Making the bread

1 piece of sour dough (about the size of a large apple)
700 ml (2¾ cups) warm water, or warm water and buttermilk
7 cups rye flour (or whole wheat or millet)
½ teaspoon vegetable salt
1 tablespoon caraway seed

Place sour dough and liquid in a warm bowl. Add half the flour and mix thoroughly, then add the remainder of the ingredients and mix well for a few minutes. Now take out a piece the size of a large apple for the next bread making session. Place the remaining dough in two greased baking tins (size of orange cake tins) or make two oval loaves and put on a floured cooking sheet, also greased. Cover with plastic bags to protect against draughts. Put in a warm place (30°C) for about 24 hours. (In summer, dough can be placed in the sun during the day.) Preheat oven to 160–190°C (350–400°F). Place bread in oven for 50–60 minutes. Cool on a rack, wrap in luncheon paper and store in plastic bag in the fridge. This bread will keep for a long time.

Scones (gluten free)

1 cup rice flour
1 cup buckwheat flour
2 teaspoons low-allergenic baking powder
1 teaspoon vegetable salt
1 tablespoon grated onion
½ cup cold pressed oil
½ cup goat's or soya milk
½ cup mashed pumpkin

Mix dry ingredients, then add herbs, onion, oil and milk. Beat well with Bamix or electric beater. Divide into twelve scones and put on sheet. Bake in hot oven for about 10 minutes.

Note:

- Scones made from other than wheat flour do not rise as well.

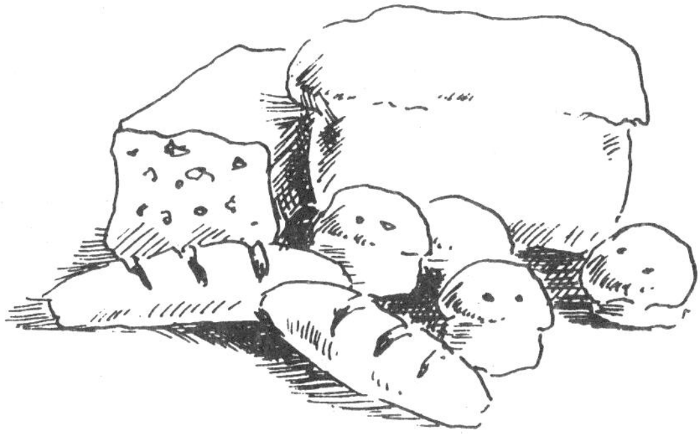

Scottish oatcakes (not gluten free)

2 cups fine oatmeal
1 teaspoon vegetable salt
¼ cup cold pressed oil
¾ cup cold water

Mix all ingredients. Roll out or press onto floured board until as thin as possible (approx. 2 mm or ⅛"). Cut into rounds and place on greased tray. Bake in hot oven for 10–15 minutes. Then turn oven down to 130°C and leave until completely cooked and dry so they can be shaken off the tray. Cool on rack covered with grease-proof paper.

Sesame crackers

½ cup melted soft butter, or oil
1 cup cold water
1 teaspoon vegetable salt (optional)
¾ cup sesame seeds (crushed in blender)
1 cup fine maize or buckwheat flour
1 cup fine millet flour
1 cup fine rice flour
¼ cup whole sesame seed

Emulsify butter, water and salt in blender. Mix into crushed sesame seeds and flour. Roll out or press, very thinly, onto greased tray. Press the whole sesame seeds into the top and cut into squares. Bake in a hot oven for 10–15 minutes. Turn oven down to 130°C and leave until completely cooked and dry, to the extent that they can be shaken of the tray. Cool on rack, covered with grease-proof paper.

Vaccination

United States Congressional hearings in 2000 and 2001 point to very serious allegations involved in the controversy over vaccination. Congressman Dan Burton, Indiana, Chairman of the Congress Committee, who has two grand-children damaged by vaccination – told of investigations by the British *Sunday Express* showing that, "... more than two thirds of the doctors and academics who serve on Committees of the Medicines Control Agency in England have investments in the pharmaceutical industry or benefit from drug company cash. Some of these doctors have huge shareholdings worth more than one hundred thousand pounds in major companies such as Smith Kline Beecham and Astrazenica. The extent of the links between the experts of the industry leaves the committees open to allegations of conflict of interest. The *Express* found 170 of the 248 members have these financial links, 42 with shares in a variety of these companies."

Congressman Burton went on to say, "We have parallel problems in America. The Chairman of the Centres for Disease Control (CDC) [who are regulatory advisors to the FDA to license the vaccines for use] until recently owned 600 shares of the stock in Merck Sharp & Dome, vaccine manufacturers, and makers of the 1998 rotavirus vaccine [that had to be taken off the market for its damage and death to children]. Four of the eight CDC advisory committee members who voted to approve guidelines for the rotavirus vaccine in June 1998 had financial ties to other pharmaceutical companies developing different versions of the vaccine. So they definitely had conflicts of interest."

The question should be asked, why do we have to vaccinate for measles? It was a 'breeze of a disease' for our grand-parents, who seem to have been healthier than we are. Everybody used to get measles, mumps and chicken-pox. Measles maybe a killer in other parts of the world, but it was not in Australia. (Except among Aboriginals, who could benefit maybe from vaccination. But Dr Kalokerinos who received an Order of Australia for his work among Aboriginal children says, "Give Vitamin C daily and measles won't worry them, either.")

Measles helps to prime our immune system. The immune system diseases have increased since measles vaccinations were introduced. (See Chapter on Treatments for ADD/HD for measures to minimise vaccination risks if you decide to vaccinate.)

UK and US findings precisely parallel

Similar findings had been made by medical doctors at the Royal Free Hospital in London, where Professor Andrew Wakefield had noted a close link between a British Government MMR vaccine campaign in 1988 and a significant rise – in fact a doubling – of autism cases. He later compared this with the steep autism rises reported in California in the 1980's and noted by way of a graph in a letter published in *The Lancet* (September 1999), the mirrored correlation to West London statistics over the same periods of times that matched the introduction of MMR vaccinations to both countries. Before this letter, Wakefield's Department of Medicine at the Royal Free had isolated vaccine measles virus in the intestines of autistic children (*Gut* 1995; 36).

The California State Department of Developmental Services (DDS) reported in April 1999 a 273% increase in autism since 1989. These figures did not include 13,500 infants to 3 year olds yet to be differentially diagnosed, who presented with neurological problems. This means a certified number of one in 312 children with autism – more, if the 13,500 includes a high percentage of autism, as the DDS reports it does, "... autism has increased dramatically over the past 11 years relative to the other developmental disabilities." The DDS reported that "... net growth in the number of persons with autism on average goes up about three times each year."

These figures have been matched by an equivalent increase in autism in the United Kingdom and in Iceland (where they have had a single authority monitoring autism for 40 years). In Great Britain "as many as 1 in 175 primary school children may suffer autism, 11 times higher than previous estimates" (*Telegraph*, London, Feb 18, 2001).

The importance of vitamin C

"If it's so good – why don't all the doctors use it?"

In 1974, the publishing house Thomas Nelson in Australia released what was to become a landmark book on vitamin C – *Every Second Child* by Australian outback doctor Archie Kalokerinos M.D. His book was later published by arrangement in the USA by Keats Publishing; it contained forewords from Linus Pauling Ph.D. and Dr Irwin Stone, President of the American Preventive Medicine Association. In his book, Dr Kalokerinos tells of Aboriginal children who were dying like flies from European diseases before his introduction of vitamin C. His work was rejected or marginalized.

However, clinical evidence began to trickle in. Back in 1969 a doctor working among Aboriginals in a community hospital in the East Kimberleys of West Australia had read an article published by Dr Kalokerinos. This was just as he was giving up hope of stopping a pattern of regular deaths among young Aboriginals. He later told his story in a letter to Archie Kalokerinos.

> "When I took up my post in the East Kimberleys, I was told by my predecessor that I could expect a high mortality rate in the Aboriginal children – this was despite the availability of all modern medication and a hospital that had reasonable facilities … it was only after losing six young patients in three months that I realised the truth of this statement … I remember sitting down with my Matron and some of the nursing staff in a state of depression discussing where we had failed and being totally unable to fault the treatments …
>
> When I read your article I was prepared to use Gorgonzola cheese intravenously if it would have any effect and so I circulated your article …
>
> Bottles of vitamin C were given at every opportunity. All in-patients below the age were given 100mg twice daily regardless of diagnosis and continued after discharge … the results were remarkable and over the ensuing nine months there were no more deaths that could not be satisfactorily explained.
>
> The nursing staff and Matron were extremely impressed …

> When I left, my successor stopped vitamin C therapy ... the result was immediate return to the old mortality."

Today, some doctors give as much as 60,000 milligrams intravenously, or even more in some cases, for certain acute diseases and also for chronic disease. According to Lady Cilento, Queensland's famous doctor of medicine (the 'Medical Grandmother' as she was affectionately known), use of vitamin C intravenously would cure meningococcal disease if used in time. She used this procedure successfully. Why isn't this used today?

Vitamin C does many things in our body, it is an essential element. Among these effects, it can help to take out (chelate) heavy metals and can also chelate chemicals.

Journey into the land of make believe

"Nearly half of all family doctors had reservations about giving children their second dose of MMR vaccine."

Adverse Reactions
November 2000; Vol 19, No. 4
and *The Sun Herald*, London, December 10
(from study of UK Welsh doctors)

Unbelievable but true – how vaccines are made

Science Report by Michael Sichel DO ND PhD

What we have been made to believe about immunisation is shattered by a close look at what really goes on behind the scenes.

A typical vaccine serum is made of basically four components:

- the targeted disease virus or other pathogen
- the cells in which the virus exists
- the fluid in which the cells live
- the chemicals that preserve the vaccine

Each of the above can cause major problems, well-known in the vaccine industry.

Because American regulatory agencies, by default, virtually govern world-wide use of vaccines you need to understand a little about these agencies, some of whom are under investigation for corruption.

Initials of the regulatory bodies involved in licensing a vaccine:

- FDA US Food and Drug Administration
- CDC The Centres for Disease Control – The 'Vatican' of world medicine
- CBER Centre for Biologic Evaluation & Research, FDA vaccine approval branch
- IOM Institute of Medicine, supposedly an independent scrutinising body

Just like the hermit crab, viruses which cause measles and mumps and other childhood problems need a 'nest' to live in and food to 'eat'. In the case of a normal infection by a human disease virus, this is a cell in the body of the host person, which provides both shelter and nutrition. Vaccine, such as the MMR vaccine, are made from live but attenuated (weakened) measles, mumps and rubella viruses which are grown in the cells of chicken embryo cells. The chick embryo becomes both the food and the home of the growing vaccine. When mature, the cells are separated and mixed with the anti-biotic preservative neomycin (other preservatives in other vaccines can include mercury, formaldehyde, aluminium) to try and maintain the attenuated state and stop cross contamination by stray pathogens that can thrive in these conditions. Other vaccines are grown in cells taken from, for instance, African Green Monkey kidney cells and fed with the serum (blood product) of calves. Because such vast quantities of vaccine are needed, scientists have developed cells that multiply by themselves. These are called 'immortal cell lines' which, like cancerous cells, keep on replicating.

In the US, Mad Cow Disease is now considered a potential problem in culturing, according to an FDA report (29 Dec, 2003).

Problems

It is common knowledge in the vaccine industry that vaccines grown in chicken cultures, like the MMR used in Australian children, are plagued with some serious viral contamination. The virol textbook *Fields Virology* (2001 edition) states: "At the present time, vaccines produced by some of the world's 12 manufacturing institutes are contaminated with avian leukosis virus."[1] Avian leukosis virus (AVN) affects large segments of the modern poultry industry, is present in commercial chickens and eggs, and we are exposed to this on a constant basis. AVN or its components still linger in both human and animal vaccines.[2,3] These components include some potentially nasty viruses, including a sarcoma (cancer) virus[4] (ALSV).

Junk genes

AVN is capable of becoming a 'parent' of other virus forms, "transforming into a dizzying array of related viruses by hijacking one of numerous cancer-related gene segments from its host, and inserting this into its own genome."[5] These genes even have a nickname in the vaccine industry –'junk genes'.

In 2001, the CDC tried to mitigate damage to the image of immunization, by publishing a study that claimed there was no transmission of the AVN viruses to MMR recipients (they did not deny the AVN was present in the vaccine). However, immunologists pointed out that given the known behaviour of ALSV, a blood serum test will not always provide correct evidence of a particular virus's presence in the human body. They advised further investigation, as the particles can retreat into the tissues, so not found in the blood.

It seems there is an unsettling lack of knowledge about viruses pumped into our children's bloodstream. In the light of an undeniable pandemic of new children's diseases this is ignorance almost of a criminal nature.

The cells in which the virus grows and other serums on which they feed

Possibly even more risky is the production of the previously mentioned immortal cell lines that keep dividing on and on (and on). Unfortunately for our children, after several hundred such divisions (called 'passages' in vaccine language) of so-called Vero cells, the likelihood of tumour production increases more and more. One study found "passage No.232 and higher produced tumour nodules in all mice inoculated."[6] (The mice used for this study had no functioning immune system, but then, some of our children have very depleted immune systems, too.)

One investigator found evidence in two studies showing that the immortal cell lines can react differently in animals of different species.[7,8] For example, cells from one species allows immortal cells to bring about cancerous changes faster than cells from another species. ***This is an ongoing concern for the vaccine industry and its regulators.*** In March 2001, the FDA sent a circular to vaccine manufacturers which said, "In general, CBER currently views Vero cells as an acceptable substrate for viral vaccines, but has residual concerns." The letter went on to warn that "all products derived from Vero cells be free of residual *intact* [author's italics] Vero cells. If your manufacturing process does not include a validated filtration process to clear residual intact Vero cells from the product, please incorporate such a procedure into your manufacturing process."[9]

Just think, for one moment, here it is – a letter written in 2001 with over 50 years of widespread vaccination behind the regulators, and still somebody is producing a questionable product! The vaccination program has always been accompanied by evidence of small or widespread reactions – e.g. officially recorded deaths of five Australian children over a 19 month period. Because adverse reactions are admitted to be less than 10%, multiply all figures by ten. Even then, most claims are denied by regulators and even

Government,[10] yet the above serious filtration request is made to manufacturers! This is a public scandal that should arouse in us anger and dread at the lies and disregard for human suffering.

As Barbara Loe Fisher, President of the US National Vaccine Information Center has commented, "Who is minding the public health when the FDA allows drug companies to produce vaccines grown on animal tissue cultures and they don't even know if this practice is facilitating cross species transfer of animal viruses into man?"

But the FDA and the CDC ***do know*** that illness linked to cross-contamination in vaccines is being found.

In early 1994, "a region of sequence homology [similar in structure] to African green monkey simian cytomegalovirus (SCMV) was noted [in a patient]" by John Martin M.D. Ph.D. of the Center for Complex Infectious Diseases, and ***reported to the CDC***.

In December 1994, Dr. Gary Hayward of Johns Hopkins University submitted additional sequence data on SCMV to GenBank. From his sequence data, it was unequivocal that the Chronic Fatigue Syndrome (CFS) patient's virus had originated from SCMV. This conclusion was ***reported to the FDA*** in March of 1995.

As infectious disease researcher Dr John Martin comments:

> "If a vaccine program were to be initiated today, one would surely not import wild monkeys from Africa, create short term primary kidney cultures, add a human virus and administer the crude gamish derived from the virally infected cells to virtually every child in the country. Nor would one want to withhold applying the many molecular biological techniques developed over the last 30 years to assess vaccine purity. Yet this is essentially the situation with live polio vaccine and comparable arguments can be made for other human and animal viral vaccines."[11]

The reality of these crude methods of vaccine preparation were made plain by Dr Martin's report of the history of what he terms 'stealth viruses'.

> "In 1991, I coined the term 'stealth' to describe the viruses that were being identified in blood and CFS (Chronic Fatigue Syndrome) cultures, and which had been seen on electron microscopy of the brain biopsy. This term was used primarily because it denoted a cytopathic infection occurring in the absence of inflammation. The SCMV-derived virus isolated from patient D.W., was designated stealth virus-1. She has remained quite disabled with fatigue and cognitive impairment. Positive cultures are still obtainable from this patient."

The fluid (culture) nutrients in which the cells live

We have discussed avian viruses in chicken embryo culture, used for measles, mumps and rubella, but the most common general vaccine nutrient used is serum from fetal calf blood. This can be loaded with all kinds of micro-organisms. In particular, bovine diarrhea virus, mycoplasma, bacteroides, nanobacteria, and a frequently found poliomegalo virus (SM40) from Green Monkeys, associated with cancer.

Although much work has been done on some of these (e.g. SM40), the complex manner in which these pathogenic particles interact is not fully known, and since the possible pathways are endless, probably never will be.

New pathogens are being found in bovine fetal serum. As molecular investigative tools improve and the molecular world comes alive to scientists, new bacteria and other pathogens are being found that would have escaped detection by vaccine regulating laboratories only a few years ago. One of these species is nanobacteria ('nano' means one-billionth, so a nanobacterium is an extremely small bacterium). How could such a tiny organism hurt us? Scientists around the world have found nanobacteria cause or are present in many major diseases, whose cause has always been questioned, such as coronary artery calcification, atherosclerotic heart disease, and all kinds of skin diseases, infectious polycystic kidney disease, and brain problems where it affects the pineal gland.

Bovine herpes viruses is also persistent in calf serum. One researcher[12] warned that his tests showed a 100 times increase of these infectious particles in calf-serum, and "since this is the first bovine human herpes and Epstein-Barr (glandular fever) related virus which replicates on human cells in the laboratory, the danger of possible human infection should not be ignored."

The list of studies of possibilities of pathogenic disease in cultures is endless.

The chemicals which preserve the vaccines

See also the attached US Congress Medical Testimony Report – autism and mercury preservative

Up until the late1990's thimerosal, preservative containing 50% mercury (Hg) in MMR vaccines and others, caused babies to be injected with 100 times the allowable (EPA) daily mercury exposure level. It is still used in some Australian vaccines.

You would probably not ask someone to inject your child with a mercury product. Prof. Boyd Haley, Chemistry Dept. Uni. Kentucky, a world expert on Hg toxicity, has stated, "Mercury is one of the most neurotoxic compounds known to man." And neurological disease is the most prevalent concern in the rapidly growing epidemic of major childhood problems. But at least one manufacturing company claimed safety for their product, thimerosal. Repeatedly, over several decades, they were sent studies from prestigious research questioning their marketing of thimerosal. These included warnings from the FDA. But it was not until the early 1990's that production ceased. However, according to legal investigators, records show they are to receive licensing royalties on its production until about 2010. So somebody, presumably, is still manufacturing thimerosal.

The above information comes from disclosure documents by law firms engaged in class actions against the company on behalf of parents with children claimed to be damaged by vaccines. Class actions in the USA got underway in 2001. Similar actions are underway in England, Scotland, Ireland and Canada.

Despite these actions and directives from the Institute of Medicine, stocks were not recalled. A national survey found about 5% of vaccine stocks still contained Hg.

Regulators deliberately altered critical study results

In 2002, one of the law firms involved with parents suing the US Government and pharma companies for autism damage to their children through neurological mercury injury, announced they had come into possession of an unreleased confidential report authored by Centers for Disease Control scientists. The report stated they had "found increasing risks of neurological developmental disorders with increasing cumulative exposures to thimerosal." The report included a graph showing a child's increasing risk with every vaccine containing mercury. ***But a different version of the report was given to the Institute of Medicine, which said the matter of vaccine preservatives was 'inconclusive'.*** Moreover, the study's chief author, Thomas Verstraeten, has since left the CDC and is now employed by GlaxoSmithKline, a manufacturer of thimerosal containing vaccines, which is facing numerous lawsuits in both America and Europe.

Other currently used preservatives are also known toxic agents. Aluminium, a heavy metal, is implicated in neurological disease. Formaldehyde has known mutagenic properties (it can change gene replication). And what other, undisclosed, preservatives are used? This is anybody's guess. For by now it has become obvious that few in the vaccine industry can be trusted.

The above sections tell about some of the concerns associated with vaccine production. Because of the 'virus-soup' being injected, there are many other possibilities, including:

- How many vaccine related sub-clinical problems lie behind the growing pandemic of **learning difficulties**?
- Does **meningitis**, now fast becoming a concern, have a vaccine damage base?
- What happens to the next generation? What **wild strains** will develop aboard a human host? This is a Frankenstein scenario. But possible.

And much more could be said of the stuff which they blandly inject into our kids.

Short extract of testimony before US Congress 2002

Autism: A unique type of mercury poisoning

Sallie Bernard, Albert Enayati, B.S., Ch.E., M.S.M.E., Heidi Roger, Teresa Binstock, Lyn Redwood R.N., M.S.N., C.R.N.P., Woody McGinnis M.D.

The characteristics of autism and mercury poisoning, derived from a review of medical literature, have been found, upon comparison, to be strikingly similar. The characteristics of both disorders are summarized in the following table and fully elucidated in the body of this document. The parallels between the two diseases are so close that it would be unreasonable to assume that the similarities occur by chance. We claim that autism is a form of mercury poisoning, based on similarities of characteristics and on the known exposure to mercury of the majority of US children. The exposure route is childhood vaccines, most of which contain thimerosal, a preservative comprised of 50% ethyl mercury by weight. The amount of mercury a typical child under two years receives from vaccinations equates to 237.5 micrograms, or 3.53×10^{17} molecules (353,000,000,000,000,000 molecules), most of which is not excreted and goes directly to the brain. The amount is known to exceed Federal safety standards, but is still considered a "low" level, such that only a small percentage of exposed individuals will exhibit signs of toxicity. Affected individuals are those genetically prone to mercury sensitivity, which is consistent with the observed high heritability rate of autism. Furthermore, the timing of mercury exposure via vaccines coincides with the emergence of autistic symptoms. Moreover, mercury has been detected in urine, hair, and blood samples from autistic children, and parental reports, though limited at this date, indicate significant improvement in symptoms with administration of standard heavy metal chelators. Thus, the four agreed-upon criteria used by clinicians to diagnose mercury poisoning – i.e., observable symptoms, known exposure at the time of symptom onset, detectable levels in biologic samples, and improvement with chelation – have been met for autism.

Comparing characteristics of autism & mercury poisoning

	Mercury Poisoning	**Autism**
Psychiatric Disturbances	Social deficits, shyness, social withdrawal	Social deficits, social withdrawal, shyness
	Depression, mood swings; mask face	Depressive traits, mood swings; flat affect
	Anxiety	Anxiety
	Schizoid tendencies, OCD traits	Schizophrenic & OCD traits; repetitiveness
	Lacks eye contact, hesitant to engage others	Lack of eye contact, avoids conversation
	Irrational fears	Irrational fears
	Irritability, aggression, temper tantrums	Irritability, aggression, temper tantrums
	Impaired face recognition	Impaired face recognition
Speech, Language & Hearing Deficits	Loss of speech, failure to develop speech	Delayed language, failure to develop speech
	Dysarthria; articulation problems	Dysarthria; articulation problems
	Speech comprehension deficits	Speech comprehension deficits
	Verbalizing & word retrieval problems	Echolalia; word use & pragmatic errors
	Sound sensitivity	Sound sensitivity
	Hearing loss; deafness in very high doses	Mild to profound hearing loss
	Poor performance in language IQ tests	Poor performance in verbal IQ tests
Sensory Abnormalities	Abnormal sensation in mouth and extremities	Abnormal sensation in mouth and extremities
	Sound sensitivity	Sound sensitivity
	Abnormal touch sensations; touch aversion	Abnormal touch sensations; touch aversion
	Vestibular abnormalities	Vestibular abnormalities

	Mercury Poisoning	Autism
Motor Disorders	Involuntary jerking movements – arm flapping, ankle jerks, myoclonal jerks, choreiform movements, circling, rocking Deficits in eye-hand coordination; limb apraxia; intentional tremors Gait impairment; ataxia – from incoordination & clumsiness to inability to walk, stand, or sit; loss of motor control Difficulty in chewing or swallowing Unusual postures	Stereotyped movements – arm flapping, jumping, circling, spinning, rocking; myoclonal jerks; choreiform movements Poor eye-hand coordination; limb apraxia; intentional movements Abnormal gait and posture, clumsiness and incoordination; difficulties sitting, lying, crawling, and walking Difficulty chewing or swallowing Unusual postures
Cognitive Impairments	Borderline intelligence, mental retardation – some cases reversible Poor concentration, attention, response inhibition Uneven performance on IQ subtests Verbal IQ higher than performance IQ Poor short term, verbal and auditory memory Poor visual and perceptual motor skills, impairment in simple reaction time Difficulty carrying out complex commands Alexia (inability to comprehend the meaning of written words) Deficits in understanding abstract ideas and symbolism; degeneration of higher mental powers	Borderline intelligence, mental retardation – sometimes 'recovered' Poor concentration, attention, shifting attention Uneven performance on IQ subtests Verbal IQ higher than performance IQ Poor short term, auditory and verbal memory Poor visual and perceptual motor skills, lower performance on timed tests Difficulty carrying out multiple commands Hyperlexia (ability to decode words while lacking word comprehension) Deficits in abstract thinking and symbolism, understanding other's mental states, sequencing, planning and organizing
Unusual Behaviors	Stereotyped sniffing (rats) ADHD traits Agitation, unprovoked crying, grimacing, staring spells Sleep difficulties Eating disorders, feeding problems Self injurious behavior, e.g. head banging	Stereotyped, repetitive behaviors ADHD traits Agitation, unprovoked crying, grimacing, staring spells Sleep difficulties Eating disorders, feeding problems Self injurious behavior, e.g. head banging

	Mercury Poisoning	Autism
Visual Impairments	Poor eye contact, impaired visual fixation	Poor eye contact, problems in joint attention
	'Visual impairments', blindness, near-sightedness, decreased visual acuity	'Visual impairments', inaccurate/slow saccades; decreased rod functioning
	Light sensitivity, photophobia	Over-sensitivity to light
	Blurred or hazy vision	Blurred vision
	Constricted visual fields	Not described
Physical Disturbances	Increase in cerebral palsy; hyper- or hypo-tonia; abnormal reflexes; decreased muscle strength, especially upper body; incontinence; problems chewing, swallowing, salivating	Increase in cerebral palsy; hyper- or hypotonia; decreased muscle strength, especially upper body; incontinence; problems chewing and swallowing
	Rashes, dermatitis/dry skin, itching, burning	Rashes, dermatitis, eczema, itching
	Autonomic disturbance: excessive sweating, poor circulation, elevated heart rate	Autonomic disturbance: unusual sweating, poor circulation, elevated heart rate
Gastrointestinal Disturbances	Gastroenteritis, diarrhea; abdominal pain, constipation, "colitis"	Diarrhea, constipation, gaseousness, abdominal discomfort, colitis
	Anorexia, weight loss, nausea, poor appetite	Anorexia; feeding problems/vomiting
	Lesions of ileum & colon; increases gut permeability	Leaky gut syndrome
	Inhibits dipeptidyl peptidase IV, which cleaves casomorphin	Inadequate endopeptidase enzymes needed for breakdown of casein and gluten
Abnormal Biochemistry	Ties up -SH groups; blocks sulfate transporter in intestines, kidneys	Low sulfate levels
	Has special affinity for purines and pyrimidines	Purine and pyrimidine metabolism errors lead to autistic features
	Reduces availability of glutathione, needed in cells and liver to detoxify heavy metals	Low levels of glutathione; decreased ability of liver to detoxify heavy metals
	Causes significant reduction in glutathione peroxidase and glutathione reductase	Abnormal glutathione peroxidase activities in erythrocytes
	Disrupts mitochondrial activities, especially in brain	Mitochondrial dysfunction, especially in brain

	Mercury Poisoning	**Autism**
Immune Dysfunction	Sensitivity due to allergic or autoimmune reactions; sensitive individuals more likely to have allergies, asthma, autoimmune-like symptoms, especially rheumatoid-like ones	More likely to have allergies and asthma; familial presence of autoimmune diseases, especially rheumatoid arthritis; IgA deficiencies
	Can produce an immune response in CNS	On-going immune response in CNS
	Causes brain/MBP autoantibodies	Brain/MBP autoantibodies present
	Causes overproduction of Th2 subset; kills/inhibits lymphocytes, T-cells, and monocytes; decreases NK T-cell activity; induces or suppresses IFNg & IL-2	Skewed immune-cell subset in the Th2 direction; decreased responses to T-cell mitogens; reduced NK T-cell function; increased IFNg & IL-12
CNS Structural Pathology	Selectively targets brain areas unable to detoxify or reduce Hg-induced oxidative stress	Specific areas of brain pathology; many functions spared
	Damage to Purkinje and granular cells	Damage to Purkinje and granular cells
	Accummulates in amygdala and hippocampus	Pathology in amygdala and hippocampus
	Causes abnormal neuronal cytoarchitecture; disrupts neuronal migration & cell division; reduces NCAMs	Neuronal disorganization; increased neuronal cell replication, increased glial cells; depressed expression of NCAMs
	Progressive microcephaly	Progressive microcephaly and macrocephaly
	Brain stem defects in some cases	Brain stem defects in some cases
Abnormalities in Neuro-chemistry	Prevents presynaptic serotonin release & inhibits serotonin transport; causes calcium disruptions	Decreased serotonin synthesis in children; abnormal calcium metabolism
	Alters dopamine systems; peroxidine deficiency in rats resembles mercurialism in humans	Possibly high or low dopamine levels; positive response to peroxidine (lowers dopamine levels)
	Elevates epinephrine and norepinephrine levels by blocking enzyme that degrades epinephrine	Elevated norepinephrine and epinephrine
	Elevates glutamate	Elevated glutamate and aspartate
	Leads to cortical acetylcholine deficiency; increases muscarinic receptor density in hippocampus and cerebellum	Cortical acetylcholine deficiency; reduced muscarinic receptor binding in hippocampus
	Causes demyelating neuropathy	Demyelation in brain *EEG*

	Mercury Poisoning	Autism
Abnormalities/ Epilepsy	Causes abnormal EEGs, epileptiform activity	Abnormal EEGs, epileptiform activity
	Causes seizures, convulsions	Seizures; epilepsy
	Causes subtle, low amplitude seizure activity	Subtle, low amplitude seizure activities
Population Characteristics	Effects more males than females	Male:female ratio estimated at 4:1
	At low doses, only affects those genetically susceptible	High heritability – concordance for MZ twins is 90%
	First added to childhood vaccines in 1930s	First 'discovered' among children born in 1930s
	Exposure levels steadily increased since 1930s with rate of vaccination, number of vaccines	Prevalence of autism has steadily increased from 1 in 2000 (1940s) to 1 in 500 (1990s)
	Exposure occurs at 0 – 15 months; clinical silent stage means symptom emergence delayed; symptoms emerge gradually, starting with movement and sensation	Symptoms emerge from 4 months to 2 years old; symptoms emerge gradually, starting with movement and sensation

ENDNOTES

1 Fields Virology, 2001 Vol I: 1103 (Lippincott)
2 Johnson E., Poultry oncogenic viruses and humans. *Cancer Detection & Prevention* 1994; 18 (1):9-30.
3 Johnson JA, Heneine W., Characterization of endogenuous avian leukosis viruses in chicken embryonic fibroblast substrates in production of measles and mumps vaccines. *J Virology* April, 2001
4 Johnson E, Overby L, Philpot R. *Cancer Detect Prev* 1995;19 (6): 472-86
5 Benjamin Mc Rearden, The Problem of Vaccine Contamination, cites Nevins JR, Cell Transformation by Viruses, in Knipe DM et al, 2001; *Fields Virology* (4th ed.) Vol 1, Ch.10, 245-283.
6 Levenbrook Is, Petricciani JC, Elisberg BL. *J Biol Standards* 1984
7 Contreras G, Bather JC, Furesz J, Becker BC. *In Vitro Cell Dev Bio* 1985 Nov.
8 Fuesz J, Fanok A, Contreraas G, Becker B. *Dev Biol Stand* 1989; 70
9 FDA, Division of Vaccines & Related Products Applications, March 12, 2001
10 An Australian Federal Health Minister said in 1997, children 'have more chance of dying from a meteorite' than from a vaccine.
11 W. John Martin, California Dept. of Health sponsored meeting on 20th Century Plagues, March 1, 1996
12 Egyed L. *J Clinical Microbiol* 1998 July; 36 (7)

Evidence of mercury and vaccine involvement

US Rep. Dan Burton asks parents for mercury damage letters

US Rep. Dan Burton is asking for letters from anyone who feels their child or family member has been injured by the thimerosal in the vaccines to write him a letter to the address below. It is important that senders address their letters with 'Personal Attn. Dan Burton Re: Vaccine Injury'.
His goal is to at the minimum have a thousand letters to take to the house floor. It is is very important to say in your letter if you are outside the statute of limitations for the current VICA (Vaccine Injury Compensation Act) rules.

Congressman Dan Burton
8900 Keystone Xing # 1050 Indianapolis,
IN 46240
Personal Attn. Dan Burton Re: Vaccine Injury

Send us a copy of your letter, too please: edit@doitnow.com

Here's one letter:

Dear Congressman Burton,

I am German and live in the USA since 2 years.
My child was vaccinated in Germany and damaged by American vaccines. (Glaxo Wellcome, former Glaxo Smith Kline, see the attached medical report for details.) Therefore I appreciate all your efforts and interventions to make this government clear what is going on here and tell them to stop the autism epidemic.

I am the first parent in Germany, who is running a lawsuit. As we have a different legislation I cannot sue the manufacturers (now), so I accused the pediatrician and the government forcing me to vaccine my child without telling me that there are totally toxic and neurologic damaging preservatives in the vaccines. So if you have supporting material for my lawsuits I would highly appreciate if you could send me everything you have to support my case in Germany.

My child was a superintelligent and normal, a very social child, who received – according to the Federal Agency for Health in Germany – 360 microgram of thimerosal with the DPT shots(3) and in addition several grams of aluminum with the MMR and Hepatitis A/B shot.

According to the hidden study of the CDC, 60 micrograms of thimerosal are enough to develop autism.

The synergism between thimerosal and aluminum as a toxic substance are meanwhile very well proven by scientists in the USA.

My child slipped into autism with nearly 3 years after the Hepatitis shot, the major culprit was given in early infancy with the thimerosal in the DPT vaccine. Since that time he was suffering from severe constipation which led to malabsorption and an autoimmune process was initiated. My child was very intelligent, could talk, sing and learn and he lost all speech and intelligence after the third Hepatitis A/B shot and slipped away from us during 1 week! It was a nightmare and it still is! I attach a CD-Rom, which you can use to show everywhere to demonstrate how a superintelligent child goes into a world of nightmare after the contaminated vaccinations.

To have autism and living with an autistic child is a nightmare. The children and the families live a hell on earth. Many parents are meanwhile bankrupt, mortgaging their houses to pay treatments for their children, which nobody wants to pay, many parents cannot stand it and get divorced.

I was Human Resources manager in a huge pharmaceutical company and I stopped my career as I have no trust in that industry anymore. We live a very stressful and lonely life since our child was damaged by the vaccines. I am a member of Childscreen (www.childscreen.org) to help to avoid and prevent autism. There are many options and nobody really listens! What a fatal mistake.

The research for a curable treatment of this disease goes totally in the wrong direction, as pharmaceutical drugs are researched, or drugs for a neurological disease are tested. This disease is an autoimmune disease and in the first place a gastrointestinal problem affecting the brain as the children's brain are starving essential nutrients as their digestive systems are damaged and not functioning properly. The children have a chance to recover if the right doctors will understand the link between heavy metals and the Gut-brain connection. This disease can only be cured with biomedical interventions and a total turn in lifestyle (American diet, nutrition environmental thinking etc.).

Sometimes I think those children are messengers to tell us: Stop with all this pollution, toxins etc. We have broken the laws of nature incredibly and we can only fix it with natural approaches and perhaps the society – not only in the USA but everywhere -have to make a big turn that our people stay healthy in this very toxic world.

My very best and thank you for all this effort.

Bettina Metz,
39 years old mother of an 7 year old autistic boy

The scene In Australia

Blatant propaganda in Australia

Measles vaccination

Some Government claims examined

Claim 1 **Vaccination caused the decline of infectious disease!**
Fact 1 **The diseases were already well in decline.**

Numerous scholars have demonstrated, using government statistics, that the decline of infectious disease and infant mortality in the industrialised countries began many decades before mass-vaccination. For instance, according to Dr. R. Taylor, in Australia "almost 80% of the reduction in infant mortality between the 1880s and the 1970s occurred prior to the 1930s." Extensive vaccination did not begin in Australia until the mid-1930s and for some diseases did not commence until the 1960s and later.

The decline of infectious disease was due to improvements in hygiene, nutrition, housing, and general living conditions. The figure below shows that most of the decline in measles deaths in Australia occurred before vaccination was introduced.

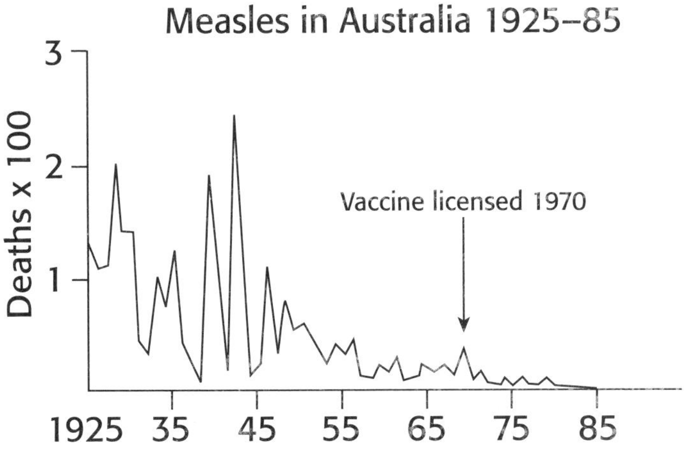

(Figure from Isaac Golden, Vaccination? A Review of Risks & Alternatives, 1994: p.4)

Claim 2 **Vaccinations are effective; only unvaccinated people get the diseases!**
Fact 2 **Outbreaks often occur in vaccinated populations.**

There are many examples in the medical literature of disease outbreaks in vaccinated populations. For example, the US Centers for Disease Control reported a measles outbreak in a documented 100% vaccinated population (*Morbidity and Mortality Weekly Report* [MMWR] 22/6/84).

In 1985, the US Government reported 1,984 non-preventable cases of measles – 80% of these were fully-immunised (MMWR 6/6/86). In 1989, of the 17,850 measles cases reported, 7,149 were appropriately vaccinated and 6,033 had evidence of previous vaccination (MMWR 1/6/90). The *Journal of the American Medical Association* (21/11/90) contains an article on measles that states, "Although more than 95% of school-aged children in the United States are vaccinated against measles, large measles outbreaks continue to occur in schools, and most cases in this setting occur among previously vaccinated children."

Note that when the media talks about 'outbreaks' they usually never mention the vaccination status of the victims.

Claim 3 **Vaccinations are safe!**
Fact 3 **The short & long-term adverse effects are not being appropriately studied.**

The reality is that no-one really knows the true extent of adverse reactions to vaccines simply because government health authorities do not make provision for, nor encourage the collection of adverse reports. It is not compulsory for doctors to report adverse reactions to vaccination. Several studies have found that adverse reactions that are noted by concerned parents are only very rarely reported by doctors. Even less are investigated by government health departments.

Documented adverse-effects of measles vaccination include: atypical measles, ataxia (loss of muscle coordination), brain damage, learning disability, retardation, aseptic meningitis (similar to polio), seizures (epilepsy), paralysis and death. Measles vaccination is highly suspected of being linked to Multiple Sclerosis, Reye's syndrome, Chronic Fatigue Syndrome, Guillain-Barre syndrome, blood-clotting disorders, juvenile-onset diabetes, autism, Crohn's disease and other serious stomach problems.

In the UK, there are presently more than 1,200 families involved in class action lawsuits against the UK government, doctors and vaccine manufacturers as a result of injuries and deaths caused by their recent measles vaccination campaign.

Claim 4 **(As of early 1998) Australia is about to undergo a measles epidemic if sufficient levels of vaccination aren't reached. (Government statement)**

Fact 4 **This is mere scaremongering. The modelling is flawed.**

The government has based their current measles campaign on mathematical modelling used by the UK government to 'predict' a similar epidemic in 1994-95. However, this ignores published medical evidence from the August 1995 issue of the *Bulletin of Medical Ethics*, which said that:

1) There was never going to be a measles epidemic in the UK – the modelling to predict it was flawed;
2) The British government knowingly misled parents about the need for the campaign and about the relative risks of measles disease and measles vaccine;
3) The Department of Health broke the European Union's law on contracts and tendering to ensure that two particular vaccine manufacturers were awarded the contract (how is Australia's vaccine contract being awarded?); and
4) The UK had a large stock of vaccine which was approaching its use-by-date. (Does Australia also have vaccine which must be used in the near future?)

Thanks to Australian Vaccination Network

Today, in Australia we are also heavily manipulated by the media. This especially applies to medical matters. In addition, Federal and State Governments appear to often sideline both effective alternative treatments and practitioners. There appears to be a nexus here with opposing international pharmaceutical companies. Australian 'health' is known world-wide to be one of the most heavily regulated with a strong and often unfair bias towards the pharmaceutical industry. Many times during my 35 years in this industry, I have seen the Government regulatory body, the Therapeutic Goods Authority (TGA), take away legitimate and *most useful* remedies, widely used in Europe or America, sometimes for centuries. It has angered me that they so blatantly allow drugs into Australia *with well known side-effects.*

One such instance is NSAID's (Non-Steroidal Anti-Inflammatory Drugs for arthritis, etc) that actually have a documented history of killing hundreds of people through internal haemorrhage[20], while natural anti-inflammatory agents have been powerfully discouraged.

In the mid-to-late 1990's, I was closely involved with others and responsible in large part, for the introduction into Australia of possibly the best natural anti-inflammatory agent there is – bovine tracheal cartilage (BTC). I visited and worked with the American surgeon John Prudden MD M.Sc, discoverer of this unique healing agent. From this work has come the wide use of chondroitin sulphate and other substances found richly in cartilage.

On returning from the States, I tried to introduce BTC to the Arthritis Foundation. With me, I had Dr Prudden's results of studies on over 700 hospital patients at the world's largest hospital – the Presbyterian-Columbia in New York. No less than 75% of these severely diseased hospital patients had almost complete remission of their pains. In some cases their joints had regenerated. Unheard of in medicine for any drug, these results were ridiculed by the Professor of a University Rheumatology Chair, to whom I had been referred by the Foundation. *This specialist, responsible for the care of thousands of people in pain, showed no interest in a new approach that came from an impeccable medical source, but was not advocated by the pharmaceutical industry, the only source he trusted.*

His only comment, "I've published more papers than Prudden." He was saying, who is this man with only 65 published papers in the medical literature?

It was at that point in time that I realised we are dealing with a system that is not dedicated to truth and open research. A system that more reflects the Dark Ages than modern science.

Right now, BTC is used widely in Australia and New Zealand, duplicating the results of the medical pioneer Dr John Fletcher Prudden, the Linus Pauling Scientist of the Year for 1996.

In 2001, the NSW State Government called for submissions on child health. I submitted the results obtained and the reasons why. I spent several unpaid days on this and sent two copies of my first book *How To Beat Hyperactivity Without Drugs.* We never received any comment, despite the obvious viability of therapy and well researched references, and the forewords and citations by respected doctors in the same field of work. And I was only one of many experienced practitioners (both medical and naturopathic) whose legitimate hard work was totally ignored.

In some cases pioneering work is pilloried, as in some mediaeval witch hunt – e.g. the Channel Nine interview with Australian scientist Dr Viera Scheibner, a world authority on vaccine damage. The media still trusts in the 'experts' – often paid by their industry backers to say 'the right thing' for their best profit.[21] Often the media is partially dependant on the company concerned for its own existence via advertising revenues.

Maybe these are some of the reasons why only 7% of British people trust the media more than Government, and few trusted the Government at all. (BBC, August 2003)

Even medical doctors who use these methods are harassed. In 2002, the NSW Government appointed a Board to 'investigate' naturopathic and functional medicine. According to some, the Board was plainly punitive towards advancing alternative methods of therapy. One board member, who had no experience in use of the advancing science of nutritional and environmental medicine had a history of pursuing individual practitioners. This Board, it seemed, was keen to keep us tightly in line.

As these events were unfolding in NSW, an interview took place on national television which highlighted the sometimes deadly mistakes that can be made in orthodox medicine, and which if they happened in complimentary medicine, would result in pursuit of the responsible person and pressure of harsh penalties or imprisonment. The interview concerned a Sydney hospital investigation for possible contribution to the deaths of eight patients through a faulty radiation technique (ABC News, July 2003). These eight people may have been among the 18,000 or so who die annually from hospital mistakes in Australia.

Other pioneering doctors whom I know, have been threatened with huge fines for using methods (however safe and effective) that simply are not yet accepted in general practice.

In America doctors offices have been raided. One famous doctor, Jonathon Wright MD LLB (a doctor of law as well as medicine), was raided by several Government uniformed men who actually held guns to the head of his receptionist while they ripped through his offices – to no avail. He still practices, with one of the largest and most famous alternative medicine clinics in America. I have met with him, when he lectured in Australia – he is a truly caring and highly knowledgeable physician. What is going on in our world?

How the orthodox establishment regards safe functional medicine therapies for ASD

A letter to the MIND Institute from a parent and a response with thanks to the Schaeffer Autism Report, free on subs@doitnow.com

Dear Dr. …

My 8-year-old son is afflicted with an autism spectrum disorder. Earlier this year his treating pediatrician referred him to the MIND Institute for an evaluation of both biomedical and cognitive/behavioural treatment interventions that might be appropriate for and beneficial to him.

In a letter dated August 22, 2002, the MIND Institute declined even to see him on the grounds that I and my spouse as his parents were seeking to have him treated with biomedical interventions that, in contrast to 'psychoactive and stimulant medications', are not 'clinically proven'.

In their stark simplicity, this statement from the MIND Institute's letter to me says more about what the MIND Institute is all about than does the entire glossy, 20-odd page Annual Report that the Institute recently issued, or than the detailed PowerPoint presentation that you gave last month at Santa Clara University. I feel obliged to offer the following thoughts in response to the fact that the only biomedical interventions that are available through the MIND Institute are psychoactive and stimulant medications, as well as to the MIND Institute's asserted justification for this state of affairs, namely, that such treatments are the only ones that are 'clinically proven'.

Although it is not entirely clear what the MIND Institute means by the term 'clinically proven', I will assume for purposes of this letter that it means supported by randomized, double-blind, clinical studies. While such studies of course represent in medical science the highest achievable standard of proof of efficacy, it is not the standard by which the medical profession by and large operates, either in practice or as a matter of law.

In California, the standard of 'medical necessity' is satisfied in significant part to the extent that the effectiveness of a particular therapy is supported by 'peer-reviewed scientific and medical evidence', which may include but is not limited to randomized, double blind studies. See California Health and Safety Code §1374.33(b)(1). As I am sure you are aware, there are numerous therapeutic approaches to the treatment of the bio-chemical imbalances and systemic disorders that frequently accompany, and may well be etiologically connected to, the complex symptomatology to which we give the name 'autism' that find broad support in peer-reviewed medical and scientific literature.

To take just a single example, I have enclosed herewith a response to the claim that 'dietary interventions' (principally, the elimination from the diet of grain [gluten] and milk [casein] proteins) in the treatment of autism are 'not proven'. There are numerous other therapeutic interventions to the treatment of autism other than 'psychoactive and stimulant medications' that find similarly abundant support in peer-reviewed medical and scientific literature.

If the MIND Institute had taken the trouble to examine our boy, it would have discovered that he presents the following clinical profile. As documented through a series of laboratory cultures of stool samples, he has a history of significant gastro-intestinal yeast (candida) overgrowths. An organic acid test of his urine reveals elevated levels of arabinose (a yeast metabolite) and below normal levels of a metabolite of glutathione, an important component of the immune system, and of uric acid. (Depressed levels of glutathione can be an indicator of heavy metal exposure.) A laboratory blood test reveals above-reference range quantities of copper and below-reference range quantities of magnesium, suggesting the presence of a metabolic disorder.

He also tests positive for neurofilament – heavy subunit brain autoantibodies, suggesting the presence of an autoimmume disorder. Laboratory tests of both blood (T3) and urine (urinary thyroxine) reveal above-normal levels of thyroid hormones. Finally, and perhaps of greatest significance, a recent urine test reveals elevated levels of both mercury and aluminum.

Is it really the position of the MIND Institute that these laboratory results reveal nothing of any therapeutic relevance to his neurological disorder, and that, in light of all available medical and scientific evidence, treatment of the biochemical imbalances and systemic disorders indicated by these results has no potential for bringing about an improvement in his condition?

The MIND Institute's double standard is also revealed by the fact that there is very little 'clinical proof' (in the sense postulated above) of the efficacy in paediatric patient populations of many if not most of the 'psychoactive (e.g., SSRIs, antidepressants, and 'atypical neuroleptics') medications' of which the MIND Institute appears to be so enamoured. Virtually none of these medications has undergone clinical trials with paediatric populations and, as a result, they almost without exception bear on their label the FDA-required notation 'Not approved for paediatric use'.

Even 'stimulant medications', as in the case of methylphenidate, are not approved for children under the age of 6. (A 'developmental paediatrician' of unassailable repute diagnosed our boy at age 3 with ADHD [not ASD] and prescribed Dexedrine for him. Not only did Dexedrine not ameliorate the conditions with which we were [and still are] struggling, it made them worse.)

Reports of the overuse, misuse, and abuse of 'psychoactive and stimulant medications' that have circulated among parents for years have become so prevalent that they have penetrated even into the inner sanctum of mainstream medical discourse. In a seminal editorial in the *Journal of the American Medical Association*, Dr. Joseph Coyle of the Harvard Medical School questions the prevalent use of psychoactive and stimulant medications in paediatric populations "since there is no clinical research on the consequences of pharmacologic treatment of behavioural disturbances of very young children". He concludes with the observation that "very young children are now increasingly subjected to quick and inexpensive pharmacologic fixes as opposed to informed multimodal therapy associated with optimal outcomes".

With about the same amount of effort as would be involved in driving to my local drugstore and buying an over-the-counter medication, I have always had the ability to obtain for our boy virtually any 'psychoactive and stimulant medication' of my choice. The last thing that he needs is yet another provider of these treatment modalities. I surmise many other parents of children afflicted with ASD lent my/their political support to the public funding with which the MIND Institute was founded precisely because it offered the hope of obtaining access to forms of treatment of this vile disorder other than those that have traditionally been, and that continue to be, readily available through conventional channels. It comes as a cruel hoax to those of us who looked forward with great anticipation to the establishment of the MIND Institute to discover that it is governed by the same philosophy of medical treatment that has so miserably failed to meet the needs of our children in the past.

If the MIND Institute continues to adhere to a policy under which it provides treatment in the form of 'psychoactive and stimulant medications' to the exclusion of all other therapeutic approaches to the treatment of ASDs, then I for one intend to do everything that I can to see to it that the public funding with which the MIND Institute is currently supported is redirected to professionals and institutions more capable of addressing the multifaceted dimensions of what can only be called a medical crisis of epidemic proportions.

John ...., Oakland, CA

Dr. X responds

Dear Mr. ...

As I understand it from your letter and from talking with the people you spoke to in our clinic, your wish was to have the MIND Institute prescribe a biomedical intervention other than psychopharmacologic agents, perhaps a casein-gluten free diet. As you were told, we do not currently have expertise in this area, nor do we have a research protocol in this area and therefore we are not able to offer you this consultation.

As you know, the mission of the MIND Institute is "to find effective treatments and ultimately a cure for autism and other neurodevelopmental disorders". The purpose of our clinic is: 1) to serve as a site to foster interdisciplinary collaboration in developing better understandings of neurodevelopmental disorders, 2) to recruit research subjects and carry out prioritized research, and 3) to serve as a high-quality, consultative resource to our community. When I listed the broad array of potential treatments for autism spectrum disorders including diet therapy in my recent talk, it was to illustrate how bewildering it is for parents and providers to choose effective treatments for a particular child when there is so little research on which to base our judgements.

We are very interested in the role of diet in exacerbating and ameliorating the symptoms of autism and other neurodevelopmental disorders and have begun to design a treatment protocol that will lead to a better understanding of which children benefit from the casein-gluten free dietary approach to treatment. We are working with the departments of paediatrics, nutrition and child psychiatry to design a double blind, placebo controlled study with 'phenotypically' well-characterized children. We are also interested in developing studies of other promising treatments that are both 'mainstream' and 'alternative' medical and psychosocial treatments.

If you would like, we will enter Samuel's name and your particular clinical interests in our research database and contact you once our casein-gluten free research protocol is approved and funded. Thank you for your thoughtful review of the literature in this area. I appreciate your passionate commitment to helping your son and hope you understand our need to keep our focus on basic and clinical research and 'traditional' consultation at this point in the development of the MIND Institute.

Director, MIND Institute

Lawsuits

For lists of lawsuits world-wide see www.vaccineinjury.org or www.athimerosalattorneyforyou.com

Typical class action preliminary statement to parents seeking redress for damage, as used by US legal firm.

> "A group of parents, whose children have all suffered brain damage from exposure to toxic mercury overdosing from childhood vaccinations, took a series of legal actions designed to put an end once and for all to mercury-laced vaccines and provide relief and hope for the millions of children who have already been exposed, suffering brain damage and autism.
>
> During the past decade, the cumulative dose of toxic organic mercury from childhood vaccines increased from five to ten fold, while the average two-year old, via a routine vaccination schedule, received more than 20 times the amount of mercury exposure than the level recommended by US EPA guidelines set to protect developing infants from brain damage.
>
> The American Academy of Pediatrics issued new guidelines in 1999 that urged utilizing only mercury-free vaccines.
>
> If you feel you qualify for damages or remedies that might be awarded in this class action please fill out the form below."

Lawsuits

The drugmaker Eli Lilly has faced at least 45 lawsuits over its role in developing and selling for more than 40 years a mercury-based preservative used in childhood vaccines and now suspected of causing autism.

Since the alarm was sounded in 1999 that mercury-based preservatives in vaccines might be linked to autism, trial lawyers have met regularly to plan their legal assaults on behalf of autistic children and their parents.

Andrew Waters, whose Dallas firm Waters & Kraus has taken a leading role in autism cases with more than 50 filed, says jurors will sympathize with plaintiffs who can show that drugmakers knowingly sold vaccines containing mercury in doses much higher than allowed under federal guidelines. He said, "It just boggles the mind [how] you inject someone, much less an 8-pound baby, with one of the most toxic substances known to man."

Military pilot challenges his vaccine

A US Air Force pilot is attempting to force the military to begin a court martial against him in an effort to highlight the plight of other soldiers who have been disciplined for refusing to take a controversial anthrax vaccine.

Lt. Col. Jay F. Lacklen said he was ready to defend himself against a court martial by claiming the vaccine has had in some lots an illegal and unsafe additive called squalene, a booster that could be in more recent lots as well. But, Lacklen said, instead of prosecuting him and facing his challenge to the vaccine, the Air Force sent him on assignment to Spain. Pilots are not critically needed there, he said.

Several lawsuits challenging the vaccine have been filed around the country. They include one by two Air Force Reserve majors from Connecticut, Russell Dingle of East Hartford and Thomas Rempfer of Suffield, against the vaccine's manufacturer, BioPort Corp. in Lansing, Mich.

In Lacklen's case, the Air Force is allowing him to avoid inoculation, but other junior officers are being disciplined. It was not immediately clear how many officers have been disciplined for refusing the vaccine.

"All military members should expect equal protection, and equal sanction, from the military legal system. This is not the case in this instance," Lacklen, 56, of Dover, Del., wrote in a complaint filed with the Department of Defense's inspector general.

The government is reluctant to fight him in court for fear of losing, Lacklen claims. Much is at stake. More than 600,000 service members have been inoculated, and the Pentagon is intent upon inoculating all 2.5 million service members eventually.

Last November, the US General Accounting Office reported that hundreds of US Air Force pilots and aircrews – who were needed for potential wartime duty in Iraq – had either left the military, transferred to non-flying duties or moved to inactive status to avoid the controversial anthrax vaccine.

About 16% of National Guard pilots and aircrew members, said the GAO, changed their status to inactive between September 1998 and September 2000.

Eighteen percent of those still assigned to or participating in a flying unit in 2000 said they wanted to leave soon, the agency said.

"I have ... painstakingly explained my position to [the Air Force]," Lacklen said, "and all I got was quack medical theories to explain away my points. I think they fear a court martial because I have the science [for a successful court case] and they do not. For instance, they have no valid explanation for how the squalene got into five lots of the first vaccine batch. They keep issuing reasons that seem plausible to a layman, but are bogus in their science."

The US Food and Drug Administration, Defense Department and BioPort have denied there are any harmful additives in the vaccine. But FDA warnings, developed from complaints by military vaccine users since 1998, state that adverse reactions are expected in 5–35% of people who take the injection. That compares with the previous expected rate of 0.2%, established in the '70s and '80s.

Lacklen filed his complaint this month against his boss, Lt. Col. Edward Poling, commander of the 326th Airlift Squadron at Dover AFB in Delaware. Defense Department spokesman James Turner referred questions on the dispute to Air Force public affairs at the Pentagon where a spokeswoman declined to comment. She said the department couldn't say anything about a preliminary matter related to the inspector general.

A Dover medical clinic ordered Lacklen to receive the anthrax shot April 15. He instead produced a letter of refusal to the clinic and to the squadron's operations officer, Lt. Col. Paul Gillis. Two days later, said Lacklen, instead of disciplining him, Poling assigned him overseas 'to avoid the issue'.

Later, said Lacklen, a second officer refused the shot, using the same letter he used, yet this more junior officer was threatened with court proceedings.

ADHD QUESTIONNAIRE

All questions are important

Today's date ______________________________

Name ______________________________

Birth Date ____________________ Age __________ M / F

Address ______________________________

____

Phone ______________________________

Fax ______________________________

Email ______________________________

Number of siblings (brothers/sisters) ____________________

The child's seniority (1st child, 2nd?) ____________________

Take time to *carefully* remember child's/adult's history in Q's below

Vaccination history ______________________________

____

____

Any noticeable connection between symptoms and vaccination? Y/N

If 'Yes' explain (e.g. can you remember any *changes* in behaviour, social contact (e.g. affection, eye contact), happiness rating, unusual habits, or loss of skills (e.g. speech, vocabulary, movement) that appeared immediately or even months post-vaccinations?

____

____

____

Sleep pattern (restless etc) ______________________________

Time to bed ______________________________

Bowel movements ☐ daily ☐ or other ______________

Consistency ☐ normal ☐ hard ☐ loose ☐ alternating (hard/loose)

Caesar birth Y/N

Breast fed Y/N If Yes, how long? ______________

Type of formula/milk used when weaning ______________

First symptoms noticed at age (e.g. born with thrush; infection at 12 months; or other problem) ______________

____

Tick following and record at what age

☐ reflux at age ______ ☐ colic at age ______

☐ skin problems at age ______ ☐ pubic infections at age

☐ ear infections at age ______ ☐ respiratory infections at age ____

☐ other at age ______________________________

Anti-biotics history & other medications

Please answer as accurate as possible and include dates/age

____

____

Using or have used: Ventolin? Cortisone? Or similar? ______________

Was child in new or refurnished and/or newly decorated bedroom (carpets, etc)? Y/N ☐ At birth ☐ At age ______

Exposed to other chemicals?

____

____

Intelligence ☐ very high ☐ high ☐ average ☐ below average

Current symptoms (include any behavourial/medical/educational opinions/diagnosis) ______________________________

____

____

Sugar cravings (excessive sugar/sweet foods demand) Y/N

Allergies noted/identified (how identified? What tests used?)

____

____

Tick any symptoms present

☐ vague ☐ poor short term memory ☐ itching ☐ restless

☐ complains of stomach ☐ irritable ☐ enuretic (wets bed)

☐ moodswings ☐ hyperactive ☐ yellow/white back of tongue

☐ has trouble getting to sleep ☐ smelly stool ☐ aggressive

☐ attention deficient (easily distracted or can't concentrate)

Mother

Tick if you ever had

☐ measles ☐ chickenpox ☐ mumps ☐ rubella

During pregnancy & birthing

☐ thrush ☐ alcohol (how much) ______________________________

☐ smoking (how many daily?) ______________________________

☐ Anti-biotics? (especially tetracyclines; chloramphenicols; gentamicin sulphanamides) ☐ omeprazole ('Losec') aspirin

☐ steroids ☐ barbiturates ☐ opioids as methadone

☐ non-steroidal anti-inflammatory (e.g. Feldene, aspirin)

☐ anti-convulsives ☐ antipsychotic drugs (list) ______________

Mercury amalgams

How many? __________ Placed during pregnancy? Y/N

Any exposure to environmental chemicals (organophosphates etc)

____

____

Infected organs

☐ tonsils ☐ gall-bladder ☐ lymph ☐ teeth

☐ Other ____

During breast-feeding

Aspirin or other analgesics Y / N

ACCURATELY OUTLINE DAILY FOOD/FLUID INTAKE *(important)*

Please use a separate sheet to list all drinks and food consumed in a typical week, including breakfast (record time), 'in between' eating/drinking, lunch (record time), 'in between', dinner (record time), before bed.

Forward the completed questionnaire with your consultation fee of AUS$45 to

Fountaindale Clinic
PO Box 5054, Chittaway Bay, NSW 2261, Australia
Phone 02 4362 2458
Int'l Phone +612 4362 2458
Email adhd-specialist@hotkey.net.au

QUICK DIAGNOSTIC CHECK LIST

In first year

Were pregnancy & delivery normal? Y / N

If not please explain.

____

____

Birth weight under 2.3 kg? Y / N

Was oxygen given in first week? Y / N

Appearance of child in first weeks after birth (tick one)

☐ pale & delicate ☐ unusually healthy looking ☐ average

Baby's health problems in first 3 months

____

____

Any reaction to ☐ bright lights/colors ☐ unusual sounds?

Does child react normally for a time, then change? Y / N

If so, when did change occur?

____

Does the child appear to be unusually intelligent? Y / N

Age 4–6 months

Does child reach out or prepare to be picked up
when you approach? Y / N

Does the child rock in the crib as a baby? Y / N

Learnt to walk alone at what age? ______________________

Which describes the change from crawling to walking?

☐ normal change

☐ little or no crawling plus gradual change to walking

☐ sudden change

☐ prolonged crawling, sudden start to walk

☐ prolonged crawling, gradual start to walk

Age 2–4 years

During first 2 years does child like to be held or was limp/passive or other? Describe.

____

____

____

Is child deaf to some sounds but hears others? Y / N

Does child hold his/her hands with strange postures? Y / N

Rhythmic rocking? Y / N

Rocking for long periods? Y / N

Does child 'look through' or 'walk through' people as though they weren't there? Y / N

Age 3–4 years

Is the child 'distant', 'in a shell'? Y / N

Is the child cuddly or affectionate between the age 2–5? Y / N

Does the child exhibit any other unusual attitudes or behaviours? Y / N

If yes, describe.

____

____

____

Age 3–5 years

Tick all appropriate boxes

- [ ] hits own head
- [ ] not co-ordinated
- [ ] 'whirls like a top'
- [ ] spins coins or jars, or other things
- [ ] has unusual skills in mathematics, or puzzles or jig-saws
- [ ] can tell day of a week a certain date will fall on

How well physically co-ordinated in running, walking, balancing climbing?

____

____

Does child line things up in precise ways
and insist they not be disturbed? Y / N

Is child fascinated by mechanical objects
(vacuum cleaner, garbage removal truck, clocks etc)? Y / N

Based on the more complete check list used by the Autism Research Institute

Recommended reading and bibliography

* Indicates text books that, in the meaning of this work, comprise both orthodox and functional medicine references of authority.

Probiotics, Natasha Trenev, Avery Publishing Group 1998

* *Healing the Hyperactive Brain*, Michael M. Lyon MD, Focused Publishing 2000

* *The Yeast Connection Handbook*, William Crook MD, Professional Books 1999

Help for the Hyperactive Child, William Crook MD, Professional Books 1991

The Yeast Connection, William Crook MD, Vintage Books 1986

Children, Fools and Pesticides, Yvonne Dolman, Prism Publishing 1990

* *Behavioural Problems in Childhood*, Viera Scheibner Ph.D, Scheibner 2000

* *Nutrition Health & Disease*, Gary Price Todd MD, The Donning Co. 1988

* *Heinerman's Encyclopedia of Fruits and Vegetables*, John Heinerman, Parker Publishing 1995

Food Is Your Best Medicine, Henry R. Bieler MD, Random House 1966

* *Double the Power of Your Immune System*, John Heinerman, Parker Publishing, 1993

* *Why Your Child Is Hyperactive*, Ben Feingold MD, Random House 1985

* *The People's Pharmacy*, Joe & Teresa Graedon Ph.D, St Martins 1996

Medical Pioneer of the 20th Century, Dr Archie Kalokerinos, Biolog. Therapies 2000

* *Pharmacological Basis of Therapeutics*, Goodman & Gillman, Macmillan 1978

* *Physician's Desk Reference*, Medical Economics Co. 1996

The Science of Eating, Alfred W. McCann, G.H.Doran NY 1919

* *Talking Back to Ritalin*, Peter Breggin MD, Common Courage Press 2000

Children's Diet Book, M.Bircher-Benner MD, Keats, 1977

Journal of National Cancer Inst., 87:110-116 January 18, 1995

Japan J. Cancer Research 78.1987, World Congress on Cancer, Sydney 1994 (Book of Abstracts)

Technical Bulletin No.671, USA Dept. of Agriculture, undated

British J. of Nutrition, Gunther, British Goat Society Year Book 1953

* *Psychodietetics*, Cheraskin & Ringsdorf Ph.D, Scarborough 1989

Not All in the Mind, Dr Richard Mackarness Psych., Pan Books 1980

* *Psycho-Nutrients*, William Vayda ND, Lothian 1992

* *Your Home and Your Health*, William Rae MD FRACS, Hartley & Marks 1988

Vaccination issues

Vaccination – Medical Assault?, Viera Scheibner, Ph.D

Vaccination – The Right Choice?, Maureen Hickman, 2000

Vaccination Roulette, Australian Vaccination Network, AVN 1998

Sen. Dan Burton's Speech, US Congress, Sept. 2000

Suggested websites *(all links work at time of writing)*

www.autism.org
Treating Autism without Drugs Dr Bernard Rimland

www.feingold.org
Food & Chemical allergy Dr Ben Feingold

www.house.gov/reform
U.S. Congressman Dan Burton

www.909shot.com
U.S. Vaccination Information

www.mercola.com
All health issues Philip Mercola MD

www.adhd-specialist.com
Michael Sichel's webpage

Other references

U.S. Centers for Disease Contol from Adverse Vaccination Event Reports, reported by Dr Baughman

Jose Saavedra MD Johns Hopkins Medical Centre, Baltimore. Probiotics and Infectious Diarrhea. *American Journal of Gastroenterology,* Vol.95. No.1. Suppl., 2000

Pornpimon Phuapradit M.D. *et al J Med Assoc. Thai* 1999. Reduction of Rotavirus Infection in Children Receiving Bifidobacteria-Supplemented Formula

Boletin de Programa National de Prevencion. Secretaria de Salud. Mexico, Vol 1 (1), August 1995

American Physicians & Surgeons Inc. Press 8, 1999 *Children under 14 are three times more likely to die or suffer disease after receiving Hep B vaccines than catch Hepatitis B.*

National Childhood Encephalopathy Study: *Report on 1000 cases of serious Neurological Disorders in infants and young children,* 1979

Vaccination – The Medical Assault on the Immune System, Viera Scheibner Phd, 1993

Behavourial Problems in Childhood – The Link to Vaccination, Viera Scheibner Phd, March 2000. Recommended reading for in-depth scholarship. Call 02 4787 8203 for a copy.

MMR vaccine linked to blood 'bruising' disorder *Archives of Disease in Childhood,* March 2001, 84: 227–229 (A British Medical Association publishing division Journal)

> The disease is *idiopathic thrombocytopenic purpura (ITP).* According to this research (carried out by the Immunisation Division of the Public Health Laboratory in London) the disease is a bleeding disorder that causes severe bruising and occurs most often within the first 2–3 weeks of MMR vaccine. It can effect the brain. Its occurrence is 1 in 22,300 doses. That equals 180 cases per 2,000,000 MMR vaccinations.

Jan Schmidt MD *Molecular Microbiology of Candida Albicans,* 2000. Cites data from *Mycoses Newsletter* summarising results from 12 sentinel laboratories in New Zealand.

Middle ear infections, acute (AOM): most children develop AOM from 6–18 months. Ear drops that contain garlic extracts may reduce pain. *Archives of Pediatric & Adolescent Medicine,* July 2001.

'The often quoted position that the relationship between diet and hyperactivity has not been proven was based on research in the 1970's. It is now time to consider the useful studies of the 1980's and 90's that clearly show a relationship.'. Joan Breakey M.AppSc., Australian dietician and researcher in *Journal of Paediatrics and Child Health*, Vol 33, 1997.

Highly recommended books and articles

Health betrayal by Eve Hillary (Synergy Books Pty Ltd. St Ives Sydney) Unmasking the corporations and their influence on Government regulators. An amazing exposure from a person herself damaged by corporate greed. evehillary@smartchat.net.au

Vaccination: the hidden truth, 2003 video, features Dr Archie Kalokerinos, Dr Viera Scheibner, Dr Mark Donohoe, Dr Robyn Cosford, Dr David Richie, Dr Isaac Golden, Dr Peter Baratosy, plus parents of damaged children and a dog breeder who sees changes in dogs after several generations of vaccination (dogs breed ten generations to a human's one, thus revealing what may happen after ten human generations of vaccinated people). This compelling video is a masterful and contemporary presentation. Available from Vaccination Information Service, PO Box 4, Turramurra, NSW 2074, Australia. Phone +61 (0)2 9144 6625

Act on truth, not fear or pressure, A very well designed 6-page brochure Contact Vaccination Information Service, PO Box 4, Turramurra, NSW 2074, Australia. Phone +61 (0)2 9144 6625

The Louise Sullivan story – An Australian nanny's nightmare by Pru Hux. How government, police and magistry 'ganged-up' to destroy an innocent person, against the evidence, to protect the pharmaceutical/ medical model/ideology.

Toxic hair analysis comparison

These two hair analysis graphs, 5 months apart, tell the wonderful story of recovery of a 7-year old girl who was given up on as a hopeless ODD & ADD case. They are typical of what we find in many ASD children and young people. This girl, Zoe, is now back to normal after her poisonous load of various heavy metals had turned her into a wild and defiant child.

The metals were chelated using simple and low cost oral medicines. These can also now be used by massage via the skin (trans-dermal).

POTENTIALLY TOXIC ELEMENTS			
TOXIC ELEMENTS	RESULT µg/g	REFERENCE RANGE	PERCENTILE 68th 95th
Arsenic	0.035	< 0.14	
Lead	3.7	< 4.0	
Mercury	0.53	< 2.0	
Cadmium	0.31	< 0.50	
Chromium	0.43	< 0.70	
Beryllium	< 0.01	< 0.050	
Cobalt	0.023	< 0.15	
Nickel	0.62	< 1.0	
Zinc	160	< 270	
Copper	21	< 70	
Thorium	< 0.001	< 0.010	
Thallium	< 0.001	< 0.020	
Barium	1.6	< 7.0	
Cesium	< 0.002	< 0.010	
Manganese	0.49	< 1.2	
Selenium	0.69	< 2.7	
Bismuth	0.011	< 0.30	
Vanadium	0.069	< 0.30	
Silver	1.8	< 0.90	
Antimony	0.11	< 0.17	
Palladium	< 0.004	< 0.010	
Aluminum	13	< 22	
Platinum	< 0.003	< 0.010	
Tungsten	< 0.01	< 0.020	
Tin	0.67	< 0.80	
Uranium	0.014	< 0.20	
Gold	0.02	< 0.40	
Tellurium	< 0.05	< 0.050	
Germanium	0.045	< 0.085	
Titanium	0.89	< 2.0	
Gadolinium	0.004	< 0.008	
Total Toxic Exposure Index			

August 4, 2004 – This is Zoe's first Toxic Hair Analysis result. It shows significant lead, mercury and cadmium. Her school behaviour record is dismal with aggression, compulsive behaviour and several expulsions. Opposition Defiant Disorder (ODD) diagnosed by a psychiatrist.

POTENTIALLY TOXIC ELEMENTS

TOXIC ELEMENTS	RESULT µg/g	REFERENCE RANGE	PERCENTILE 68th 95th
Arsenic	0.026	< 0.14	
Lead	6.0	< 4.0	
Mercury	1.4	< 2.0	
Cadmium	0.46	< 0.50	
Chromium	0.52	< 0.70	
Beryllium	< 0.01	< 0.050	
Cobalt	0.039	< 0.15	
Nickel	1.3	< 1.0	
Zinc	220	< 270	
Copper	130	< 70	
Thorium	0.001	< 0.010	
Thallium	0.001	< 0.020	
Barium	1.6	< 7.0	
Cesium	< 0.002	< 0.010	
Manganese	0.81	< 1.2	
Selenium	0.74	< 2.7	
Bismuth	0.010	< 0.30	
Vanadium	0.14	< 0.30	
Silver	7.5	< 0.90	
Antimony	0.047	< 0.17	
Palladium	0.011	< 0.010	
Aluminum	12	< 22	
Platinum	< 0.003	< 0.010	
Tungsten	< 0.01	< 0.020	
Tin	0.23	< 0.80	
Uranium	0.007	< 0.20	
Gold	0.05	< 0.40	
Tellurium	< 0.05	< 0.050	
Germanium	0.034	< 0.085	
Titanium	0.40	< 2.0	
Gadolinium	< 0.001	< 0.008	

January 20, 2005 – After five months of chelation, numerous potentially toxic metals have significantly increased in the hair result. Yet, this 7-year old girl, previously expelled from school for defiance, bullying, class disruption and ADD (typical results of lead and mercury), is now a shining example of exuberant health and behavior. Her body is now expelling the toxic metals that caused her own expulsion. Her teachers are amazed at the change, as are her extended family and friends.

End notes and references

1 The list includes these syndromes: ADHD, ADD, Retts, Childhood Disintegrative Disorder (CDD), Aspergers, Pervasive Developmental Disorder (PDD), Landau-Kleffner, Oppositional Defiant Disorder (ODD), Smith-Magenis, Wilsons and many sub-groups called Not Otherwise Specified (NOS).

2 Centres for Disease Control (CDC), the American Government disease tracking organisation

3 Dr Bernard Rimland *The Autism Research Review International* Vol 8:2, 1994. Rimland cites books by nine sets of parents who had fully diagnosed and fully recovered children..

4 Risperidone information sheet in package warns that once a patient is feeling better they must continue the dosage to prevent symptoms from returning. This could mean a patient who's 3 or 6 or 10 is on a lifetime commitment to a medication significantly equal to having breakfast daily. *Archives of Pediatrics and Adolescent Medicine* (April 2003) reported the use of psychotropic drugs by US children more than doubled during the 1990's. This now almost matches adult usage.

5 Sometimes, but rarely, we recommend brief use of a dexamphetimine to help a child calm while the treatment takes hold. This is only for a violent, totally out-of-control child.

6 Dr Tim Buie, pediatric gastroenterologist *Report of study of 600 autistic children* Harvard University and Massachusetts General Hospital collaborative study, 2002

7 *The genetics of autism: four large-scale studies find no answers* Autism Research Review International Vol 14:1 2000 Editor: Bernard Rimland Ph.D

8 Studies have shown that some genes are 'associated' but not necessarily the primary cause. Genes play a role in some families. Environment can cause gene changes. (Rodier 2000) Smalley et al 1988; Bailey et al 1995; Folstein and Rutter 1977; Steffenburg et al 1989. *DNA Sciendes* 2003

9 DNA Sciences *Genetics of Autism* DNA.com

10 "Most believe that our genes control our health and life. That simply is not true. It is not the genes themselves that control us but rather the activation or expression of our genes that makes

the difference. Fortunately, the expression of our genes can be modified by our lifestyle and emotional balancing." Dr Joseph Mercola, Newsletter www.mercola.com 2003

11 'There is increasing evidence that physical and chemical stresses to the cell, such as heat shock, chemical poisons and viral infections, tend to activate *Alu* elements. The resultant gene reshuffling may be responsible for a variety of chronic diseases' Dr Mae-Wan Ho (*Dynamic Genomics* Lecture Series by International Society of Science in Society)

12 "*Alu* elements, are retrotransposons that move and multiply by being transcribed into RNA, then reverse transcribed into DNA copies that jump into new sites. New research is suggesting that *Alu* elements may help create new proteins from existing ones. The reasons the human genome contains so few genes – the latest count is just under 25 000, is that more than half the genes are interrupted and subject to alternative splicing." Dr Mae Wan Ho, I.S.I.S. 2003

13 V. K. Singh Ph D, Immunotherapy for Brain Diseases and Mental Illnesses, *Progress in Drug Research*, vol. 48, 1997, pp. 129-146)

14 Michael Sichel DO ND, Study of 57 ASD children, 2001

15 Statistics from various pediatric sources & Autism Research Institute

16 Dr Ford-Jones, Chief Pediatrician, Hospital For Sick Children, Toronto University, Canada

17 *Trust Us, We're Experts!*(2001) and *Toxic Sludge Is Good for You! (2000)* Penguin

18 Editors of : *Annals of Internal Medicine; J.Am Med A; New England Journal of Medicine; Canadian Medical Association Journal; Journal of the Norwegian Medical Association; The Lancet; MEDLINE/Index Medicus; New Zealand Medical Journal*; Norwegian Medical Association; *Dutch Journal of Medicine*); *Annals of Internal Medicine; The Medical Journal of Australia; Western Journal of Medicine.*

19 J.Am.Med.Assoc. Feb 2, 1981. "66% of pediatricians and obstreticians refused vaccination." Later, 1994 one third of doctors (Archives Ped. & Adol Med.)

20 The Canadian Medical Journal, in 1998, said that NSAID's killed more Canadians annually than guns.

21 *Trust Us, We're Experts!* Sheldon Rampton and John Stauber, Jeremy P.Tarcher/Putnam NY ISBN 1-58542-059-X available from Dymocks Books in Australia

22 ibid.
23 Rogers vs Whitaker (1992) Australian High Court decision.
24 Dr. Richard Moskowitz graduated Phi Beta Kappa from Harvard University and received his medical degree at New York University. He studied homeopathy in Athens, Greece and taught at the National Center for Homeopathy in Washington, D.C.
25 Bowel Finding Suggests Autism Is Autoimmune Disorder. Researchers from England have shown that unexpected bowel abnormalities in children with regressive autism may have a basis in autoimmunity. The abnormalities were distinct from previously reported conditions, pointing to the gut epithelium as a target of a specific immune response. Researchers: Centre for Paediatric Gastroenterology, with the Inflammatory Bowel Disease Study Group, Royal Free & University College Medical School, London, UK; The IBD Research Unit, St. Mark's Hospital, Harrow, London, UK, et al (2002)
26 Dr Archie Kalokerinos and pathologist Dr Glen Dettman studied the Fijian vitamin C intake from fruits etc. They found the Fijians vitamin C natural intake was 2000 mgms daily.
27 Miller (1964)
28 Viera Scheibner Ph.D. *Vaccination (1993)*
29 "The marginal advantages of the (DPT) vaccine in children over one year of age have to be offset against adverse effects of the vaccine itself, which are very common indeed and may be followed occasionally by irreversible brain damage, paralysis and mental deficiency. Because of this danger, or for fear of it, many parents and doctors are reluctant to vaccinate their children. Despite the reassurances of their advisers, the Government shares this fear and has offered compensation to any children shown now or in the past to have suffered brain damage from this (or any other) vaccine." Prof. Gordon Stewart member Expert Committee U.K Government Safety of Medicines (1982)
30 Ronne (1985) found evidence of a relationship between lack of rash in measles and increased incidence of degenerative and autoimmune diseases. As cited by Viera Scheibner Ph.D. *Vaccination* p.83. (1993)
62 See www.hacres.com or *God's way to ultimate health* by Dr George Malkmus, Hallelujah Acres, P.O. Box 10, Eidson TN 37731
31 Dan Med Bull 1988 Apr;35(2):185-7
Prevalence of IgG-antibodies to mumps and measles virus in non-vaccinated children.

Glikmann G, Petersen I, Mordhorst CH. Ornithosis Dept, Statens Seruminstitut, Copenhagen, Denmark.
The prevalence of mumps and measles IgG antibodies in a randomly selected population of children was determined by an enzyme-linked immunosorbent assay (ELISA) **before routine measles-mumps-rubella (MMR) vaccination was introduced in Denmark**. Testing of sera from about 2,520 Danish children between one and 17 years of age showed that mumps antibodies were acquired at an early age. The peak acquisition rate was between the ages of four and five; before the age of 15, 90% of children had antibodies to mumps. Immunity to measles occurred at an even earlier age; more than 50% of four-year-old and nearly all (98%) nine year-old children had IgG antibodies to measles virus. The study showed that about 10% of the young adult Danish population was still susceptible to mumps infection whereas only about 1% of individuals at age 17 had not acquired immunity to measles virus.

32 "Wakefield et al. are to be congratulated on opening yet another window onto the ever-broadening spectrum of gut-brain interactions. Their findings raise many challenging questions that should provoke further much-needed research in this area, research that may provide true grounds for optimism for affected patients and their families." *American Journal of Gastroenterology Editorial*, September 2000: Volume 95, Number 9; pages 2154-2156.

33 US Special Education Stats (2000) of 5 categories of learning, emotional and autism-type disabilities.

34 This vaccine alert was revealed as a scandal by the British *Journal of Medical Ethics*, whose Editor, a pediatrician, showed the Health Ministry to have deceived the population into believing a measles epidemic was imminent. As a result 7 million English school children received the MMR shot. Following this, hundreds of cases of ASD occurred. The reason for the false alarm? The vaccine company sought Government help to dispose of approaching 'Use by Date' stocks. *J.Med Ethics* commented "you cannot trust Government doctors".

35 Epidemiology. Autism Studies: Why parents of children with autism are so upset! F. Edward Yazbak, MD. www.autismautoimmunityproject.org/upset.html.
Anti-Wakefiled studies:
The Peltola Studies were funded by Merck & Co. **The Taylor Studies** were commissioned by the Medicines Control Agency

of the UK Department of Health. **The Kaye Study**. James A Kaye, epidemiologist, the Boston Collaborative Drug Surveillance Program. Supported by grants from AstraZeneca, Berlex Laboratories, Boehringer Ingelheim Pharmaceuticals, Boots Healthcare International, Bristol-Myers Squibb Pharmaceutical Research Institute, GlaxoWellcome, Hoffmann-La Roche, Janssen Pharmaceutica Products, R W Johnson Pharmaceutical Research Institute; McNeil Consumer Products, and Novartis Farmaceutica.

36 Congressman questions officials at thimerosal hearings 06/20/2002 VALERI WILLIAMS / WFAA-TV
... research showed that the FDA began asking questions about the dangers of thimerosal back in 1972. By 1992, the preservative was pulled from dog vaccines and contact lens solutions, because of risks. Sen. Dan Burton, Chairman of the Committee, called for criminal penalties for any government agency that knew about the dangers of thimerosal in vaccines, and did nothing to protect our children.

37 Press release: Waters & Kraus, Texas law firm. Media enquiries on US number +1 214 226 6244.

38 US Congressional hearings: 2001–2002, numerous scientific presentations.

39 M. Kielinen et al, in a study published in the Journal of European Child & Adolescent Psychiatry described a significant rise in autism in the northern provinces of Oulu and Lapland, which represent 1/8 of the total population of Finland. The Kielinen study included all children born in the two provinces, between 1979 and 1994. Every single one of those children was eligible and must have received the MMR vaccine. The authors personally reviewed all records of children with autism to determine that they fulfilled the criteria. The cumulative incidence of autism was 12.2/10,000, a significant increase when compared to the previously reported incidence of 4.75/10,000 by Vinni and Timonen. The increase in the younger children, all born in the second half of the MMR campaign, was even more striking. In the 5 to 7 age group, the cumulative incidence was 20.7/10,000 or more than 1 in 500.

40 Stockholm, Sweden, (2003) In June the Swedish Dental Material Commission released a report recommending dental mercury amalgam be banned. Chief scientist: Professor Emeritus Maths Berlin. His risk anlaysis was based on science published between 1997-2002 and current knowledge. Berlin had previously led two World Health Organization Task Group –

one on inorganic mercury and one on methylmercury. He also testified before the US Congress Subcommittee on Human Rights and Wellness on May 8, 2003.

42 Waters & Kraus (ibid.)

43 *Genuine immunity versus vaccine immunity* Moskowitz, Richard, M.D. New York University & Harvard University. 1985

44 In Australia, mercury was taken from MMR vaccines about 2001, but kept in many other vaccines.

45 Autism Research Institute Pub. April 2003 Editor: Dr Bernard Rimland

46 Aderbal Sabra, JosephA Bellanti, Angel R Colón International Center for Interdisciplinary Studies of Immunology, and Department of Pediatrics,Georgetown University Medical Center, Washington, DC 20007, USA

47 Bernard Hube Ph.D. Uni Hamburg Dept Mycology 1998. *J Mycology*

48 Kretschmar M at al, *Mycoses* 1999 Vol 42 *C.albicans* "able to reach the brain and germinate in both kidneys and brain."

49 Dr John Tintera (1969) Sugar causes hyperactivity via hyperadrenaline production

50 N.Serguett et al *American Association of Osteopathy Jounral* (Spring, 2001)

51 J Child Neurol 2002 Sep;17(9):700-2 Fiumara A, Polizzi A, Mazzei R, Conforti L, Magariello A, Sorge G, Pavone L. Department of Pediatrics, University of Catania, Italy.

52 AOM or acute otitis media is considered a 'super-infection' – one that follows antibiotic failures. Harrisons' *Principles of Internal Medicine*

53 The age of onset of symptoms has changed over the years. Figures from the Autism Research Institute Database, the largest anywhere, clearly show that earlier, most parents in the USA noticed autistic behavior shortly after birth and in infancy (Kanner's infantile autism) while after 1980, 66% of parents report that their children's autistic symptoms started at or after 18 months of age (late-onset or regressive autism).

55 Myelin is the sheath or covering found around nerve fibres. It acts like the black, yellow or green plastic that covers an electric wire. It is made principally of phospholipids (lecithin).

56 Dr Tim Buie, pediatric gastroenterologist, team leader, Harvard University/Massachusetts General Hospital collaborative study Project 2002

57 "Further work thus clearly needs to be done to determine the role of the 'gut-brain axis' in autism. However, confirmation

that autoimmune responses really do contribute to cognitive regression in autistic children will raise the probability of a fundamental change in the treatment of autistic regression, based on modulating the immune response in children with early autistic symptoms." Autoimmunity in Autism, by J Licinio, I Alvarado, and Ma-Li Wong, *Molecular Psychiatry* 2002 Volume 7:4, p.329.)

58 In Appendix V, evidence will be given of strong attempts made by Governments around the world, together with their 'buddies', the pharmaceutical companies to deny the damage and misinform the public.

59 Max Planck Institute of Psychiatry, Kraepelinstrasse 10, 80804 Munich, Germany. jbrunner@mpipsykl.mpg.de Pharmacopsychiatry 2002 Jan 35(1):1-5

60 Stated, precisely, in a letter I have read, from a Professor of Pediatrics to a G.P. colleague

61 Vera Scheibner Ph D *Vaccination* 1993 cites Bernier et al (1982); Walker et al (1987); Coulter & Fisher (1991) plus her own studies with scientist Leif Karlsson

62 "The antibody to this antigen was found in 83% of autistic children but not in normal children or siblings of autistic children. Thus autistic children have a hyperimmune response to measles virus, which in the absence of a wild type of measles infection might be a sign of an abnormal immune reaction to the vaccine strain or virus reactivation." Singh VK, Jensen RL. Department of Biology and Biotechnology Center, Utah State University, Logan, Utah, USA April 2003

63 Rindsor, W., Cheraskin, E. and Ramsay, R., *Sucrose Neutrophilic Phagocytosis and Resistance to Disease,* Dental Survey, 52,12 1976 46-48

64 Caccaro, Ruth L. and Stamle, J. *Diabetic Care,* 15, No.10, October 1992

65 Kruis, W., Forstaier, G., Scheurlen, C. and Stellaard, F. *Effects of diets low and high in refined sugars on gut transit, bile acid metabolism and bacterial fermentatiom,* Gut 32,1991,pp.367-370

66 *Candida Species & Virulence,* 1994

67 *Journal of Advanced Medicine,* 1994 7(1): 51-58

71 Dr Michael Wooldridge, interviewed by Ray Martin on *A Current Affair* – TV Feb 6, 1997

81 "Uncomplicated fever, when allowed to run its course, may be associated with some discomfort, but is not dangerous. It is actually part of the body's immune response that fights bacteria

and viruses." Mark B. Levin, M.D. and Timothy Patrick-Miller, M.D. The Pediatric Group, P.A., Princeton

82 US Congress Committee Chairman Senator Dave Weldon, letter to the Director of Centres for Disease Control (CDC), Dr Julie Gerberding, Oct 31, 2003.

83 One of the conundrums of autism is that there is an approximate ratio of four boys to every girl who gets this disease. Dr. Lovell therefore tested the possibility that it could be hormone related. The latest results were quite marked in their effects. Neurons that were pre-incubated with estrogen demonstrated substantial protection against thimerosal-induced neuron death. In contrast, the addition of testosterone caused a very large increase in thimerosal-induced neuron death. A low nanomolar level of thimerosal that gave less than 5% neuron death in three hours could be increased to 100% cell death by the addition of one micromolar level of testosterone.

Testosterone alone at this level also showed less than 5% cell death. The opposing effects of estrogen and testosterone may explain the gender-based four-to-one ratio.